Third Edition

A PRACTICAL GUIDE TO PHARMACEUTICAL CARE

A Clinical Skills Primer

Notices

Advances in science mean knowledge of drug therapy and pathophysiology changes daily. Although the authors have made every attempt to be accurate and current in the case studies, descriptions of disease states, and pharmacotherapeutics discussed in this book, readers are cautioned to consult with an expert or the scientific literature before using any of the clinical recommendations made here to provide care to their patients.

The authors and publisher have made every effort to ensure the accuracy and completeness of the information presented in this book. However, the authors and publisher cannot be held responsible for the continued currency of the information, any inadvertent errors or omissions, or the application of this information. Therefore, the authors and publisher shall have no liability to any person or entity with regard to claims, loss, or damage caused or alleged to be caused, directly or indirectly, by the use of information contained herein.

The inclusion in this book of any product in respect to which patent or trademark rights may exist shall not be deemed, and is not intended as, a grant of or authority to exercise any right or privilege protected by such patent or trademark. All such rights or trademarks are vested in the patent or trademark owner, and no other person may exercise the same without express permission, authority, or license secured from such patent or trademark owner.

The inclusion of a brand name does not mean the authors or the publisher has any particular knowledge that the brand listed has properties different from other brands of the same product, nor should its inclusion be interpreted as an endorsement by the authors or the publisher. Similarly, the fact that a particular brand has not been included does not indicate the product has been judged to be in any way unsatisfactory or unacceptable. Further, no official support or endorsement of this book by any federal or state agency or pharmaceutical company is intended or inferred.

Third Edition

A PRACTICAL GUIDE TO PHARMACEUTICAL CARE

A Clinical Skills Primer

John P. Rovers, PharmD, BCPS
Associate Professor
Drake University
College of Pharmacy and Health Sciences
Des Moines, Iowa

Jay D. Currie, PharmD
Professor (Clinical)
The University of Iowa
College of Pharmacy
Iowa City, Iowa

American Pharmacists Association
Improving medication use. Advancing patient care.

APhA

Washington, D.C.

Acquiring Editor: Julian I. Graubart
Senior Project Manager: Vicki Meade, Meade Communications
Managing Editor: Paula Novash
Graphic Designer: Michele A. Danoff
Proofreader: Amy Morgante
Indexer: Suzanne Peake

APhA was founded in 1852 as the American Pharmaceutical Association.

Published by the American Pharmacists Association
1100 15th Street, NW, Suite 400
Washington, DC 20005-1707
www.pharmacist.com

To comment on this book via e-mail, send your message to the publisher at
aphabooks@aphanet.org

Library of Congress Cataloging-in-Publication Data

Rovers, John P.
  A practical guide to pharmaceutical care : a clinical skills primer / John P. Rovers,
  Jay D. Currie. — 3rd ed.
    p. ; cm.
  Rev. ed. of: Practical guide to pharmaceutical care. 2nd ed. c2003.
Includes bibliographical references and index.
  ISBN-13: 978-1-58212-104-8
  ISBN-10: 1-58212-104-4
  1. Pharmacy—Practice. I. Currie, Jay D. II. American Pharmacists Association. III. Title.
    [DNLM: 1. Pharmaceutical Services—organization & administration. 2. Delivery of
Health Care—methods. QV 737 P8949 2007]

  RS100.3.P73 2007
  615'.1068—dc22

                                                                    2007002723

HOW TO ORDER THIS BOOK

Online: www.pharmacist.com
By phone: 800-878-0729 (from the United States and Canada)
VISA®, MasterCard®, and American Express® cards accepted.

Dedication

Readers familiar with previous editions may have noticed that three of the editors seem to be missing. Although their names may not be visible, their enthusiasm, their wisdom, and their friendship continue to permeate the book. We dedicate this edition of the Practical Guide *with sincere thanks to our friends and colleagues: Harry Hagel, RPh, MS; Randal McDonough, PharmD, MS; and Jenelle Sobotka, PharmD.*

Contents TOC

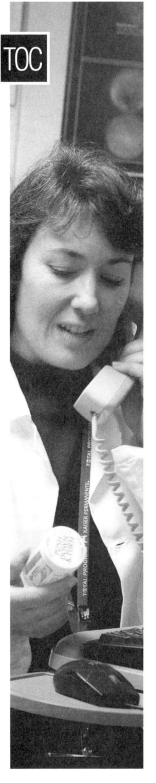

Preface 3e

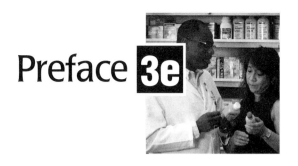

I t has been said that no man (or pharmacist) can serve two masters and it seems that books are no exception to the rule. Since the first edition of this book in 1998, our goal has been to assist pharmacists to change their practices and embrace the patient-centered practice of pharmaceutical care.

To help pharmacists undertake this daunting task, both previous editions taught pharmacists the hands-on patient care skills necessary for pharmaceutical care practice. To use these skills to their best effect, however, the pharmacy itself needs to be organized with the workflow patterns, staffing levels, marketing efforts, billing tools, infrastructure, and quality assurance programs necessary to support a practice change. Therefore, about half of our previous editions focused on these necessary tools. This was our attempt to serve two masters: practice skills and practice settings.

In this our third edition, we have gone "back to our roots" and our focus is entirely on the patient care skills that pharmacists need to provide pharmaceutical care. And, since most of our readers are student pharmacists in colleges of pharmacy in the US and elsewhere, many of the changes in this edition are designed with the student in mind. As you read through this book, we hope you will approve of the following changes:

- We have provided a list of key concepts at the beginning of each chapter. Readers who are only beginning to learn a new subject often have trouble distinguishing between what information is "need to know" and what is "nice to know." We have pointed out those sections of a chapter that are "need to know."

- Each chapter contains numerous self assessment opportunities. Pharmaceutical care looks fairly easy, and indeed it's not difficult to understand the major concepts. Often, though, it's not until it comes time to try and apply skills you have only read about that you realize you did not quite understand what you were expected to do or how to do it. We urge readers to take the self assessment opportunities we provide seriously. Try and answer each question fully before turning to the end of the book to check your answers. We've tried to provide fairly detailed ones that will help you learn how experts think about and approach this kind of practice.

- There are four new chapters in Part II of the book, Skill Application in Practice. In previous editions, the focus was entirely on pharmaceutical care practice in community pharmacy.

We have tried to expand this focus in all chapters, but have most explicitly done so in Chapters 7 to 10. In these chapters, we discuss different practice environments, including community pharmacy, hospital, long-term-care and ambulatory clinic. Each practice environment is described briefly in order to provide you with a basic notion of what pharmaceutical care opportunities may exist there. Each chapter then allows you to work up two comprehensive patient care cases set in that environment. You will need to gather history, identify problems, determine goals for therapy, design and implement a care plan, and document the care you provided.

Although none of us ever truly stops being a student, we hope this new edition will be beneficial for all student pharmacists seeking to enter a world in which patient care is a reality. If this book provides you with some of the tools to help you help your patients, then our work will have been entirely worthwhile.

John Rovers
Jay Currie

September 2006

Acknowledgments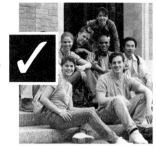

We would like to thank our students at Drake University and the University of Iowa for their assistance in telling us how they use this book and how best we could improve it. We hope our changes meet with their approval.

Contributors

Jay D. Currie, PharmD
Professor (Clinical)
The University of Iowa
College of Pharmacy
Iowa City, Iowa

John P. Rovers, PharmD, BCPS
Associate Professor
Drake University
College of Pharmacy and Health Sciences
Des Moines, Iowa

CoraLynn B. Trewet, MS, PharmD
Assistant Professor (Clinical)
The University of Iowa
College of Pharmacy
Iowa City, Iowa

Part I

Practice Skills

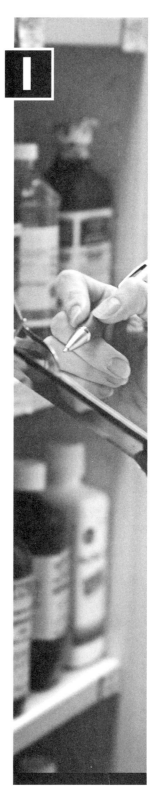

The six chapters that make up Part I of this book focus on the patient care skills a pharmacist must have to deliver pharmaceutical care. In addition, they examine what pharmaceutical care *really* means.

The True Meaning of Pharmaceutical Care

In the 17 years since Hepler and Strand first defined the term "pharmaceutical care" (see Table 1-2, page 6), its meaning has blurred. Now, when pharmacists refer to pharmaceutical care, they often mean "anything that does not include dispensing." Chapter 1 focuses on the philosophies that underlie pharmaceutical care and clarifies the modern meaning of the term. Chapters 2 through 6 detail each component of the pharmaceutical care process.

Assess Your Understanding and Practice Key Skills

At the end of each chapter in Part I, you will find self assessment questions that help reinforce key concepts from that chapter. Be sure to work through each question to derive the greatest benefit from this book. Once you have completed each question, you can check your responses in the "Answers" section at the back of the book.

The self assessments also provide good ideas to consider as you interact with patients. Try to use the concepts as often as possible. Soon they will become seamless, as well as valuable, additions to your pharmaceutical care practice.

The Case for Pharmaceutical Care

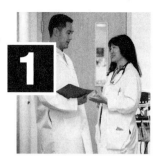

Jay D. Currie

J anice has diabetes. Her local pharmacy has filled her pre-scriptions for various oral diabetes medications for the last 5 years. Today she gave the pharmacist a prescription for Humulin 70/30, 35 units every morning. She is also currently being treated for glaucoma and hypothyroidism. She gets most of her other medications by mail order.

Edith called the pharmacy when she got home from picking up a new prescription. The directions for the medication are to take one-half of a tablet daily, but due to her arthritis she is unable to break the tablets.

George is admitted to the hospital by his primary care physician for an exacerbation of his congestive heart failure. This physician manages most of George's medical problems, but George has self-referred himself to two other physicians who are also prescribing treatment. On admission George's wife informs the primary care physician about several medicines prescribed by the other physi-cians. On the list George's wife provides is a medication known to cause control issues in patients with congestive heart failure.

Mary calls the pharmacy asking for assistance. She will shortly need to receive all her medications via a tube placed in her stomach and she wants to know which ones she can crush to get down this tube.

In each of these real-life cases, the clinical situation of a patient requires action. Depending on the care setting, the pharmacist might be the front-line health professional charged with assisting the pa-tient to resolve the problem. So what is the pharmacist's responsibil-ity to these patients? What should he or she do?

The pharmacist has a number of choices. She can ignore the situation as it is really between the patient and physician. She can instruct the patient or caregiver to discuss the problem with the physician. She can acknowledge the problem and be empathetic but do nothing to intervene. She can attempt a quick fix with some counseling or a phone call to the physician, but not offer a solution. Or she can find out what is really going on, pinpoint the apparent or unidentified problems that may exist, and work with the patient and his or her physician to make sure appropriate care is rendered and the patient achieves the desired effect from treatment.

The choices above relate to addressing a current problem. But what could a pharmacist have done in the past to minimize or even avoid that problem? Providing pharmaceutical care involves not only identifying and resolving problems that exist, but also identifying and preventing potential problems.

Adopting a New Philosophy

★ Providing pharmaceutical care means adopting a philosophy of practice where pharmacists work with and for the patient to optimize the outcomes of medication therapy. Just because a patient does not ask the pharmacist about an issue or problem, it cannot be assumed that one does not exist. Pharmacists assess the patient and the patient's medications to understand the current status and act on the patient's behalf. They take it as their duty to make sure that everything is happening in the best interest of the patient, regardless of the practice setting.

Pharmacists must not only embrace this philosophy to provide pharmaceutical care, but also create a work environment that allows it. A conceptual model proposed by Bernard Sorofman, shown in Table 1-1, suggests the changes necessary in both the pharmacy and the pharmacist to allow organized delivery of pharmaceutical care in any pharmacy practice setting.

TABLE 1-1

Systems in Place vs. Lack of Systems

		Pharmacy Site	
		Pharmaceutical care support systems in place	No support systems in place
P h a r m a c i s t	Pharmaceutical care activities	Ideal pharmaceutical care	Incomplete pharmaceutical care
	No pharmaceutical care activities customary	Expensive usual and customary dispensing with inadvertent pharmaceutical care	Usual and customary dispensing

Source: Sorofman BA. Iowa City, IA: The University of Iowa College of Pharmacy. Used with permission.

A PRACTICAL GUIDE TO PHARMACEUTICAL CARE: A Clinical Skills Primer

Pharmacists use their knowledge and skills to benefit their patients by providing ongoing care over time.

Some basic beliefs that are important to pharmaceutical care practitioners are:

• Patients need and deserve excellent care.

• Pharmacists have more to offer patients than the safe delivery of medications. They can help bring about long-term benefits to patient health.

• Pharmacists as individuals should provide personalized, direct care to patients.

This level of caring for and working with the patient goes well beyond the traditional pharmacist–patient interaction, and exceeds the training received in pharmacy school for all but the most recent pharmacy graduates. This type of pharmaceutical care goes hand-in-hand with a "reprofessionalization" of the pharmacy profession and can be thought of as the pinnacle of what pharmacists have to offer patients in the health care system.

From Products to People

In a 1986 editorial titled *Drugs Don't Have Doses—People Have Doses!*[1] Robert Cipolle defines the role of the pharmacist as a "clinical problem solver," foreshadowing the change from a product-oriented to a patient-oriented profession. In 1990, Charles Hepler and Linda Strand provided the current working definition of pharmaceutical care: "The responsible provision of drug therapy for the purpose of achieving definite outcomes that improve a patient's quality of life"[2] (see Table 1-2). Since then the American Pharmacists Association (APhA) and the American Society of Health-System Pharmacists (ASHP) have embraced this definition as the core of their *Principles of Practice for Pharmaceutical Care* and *Statement on Pharmaceutical Care*, respectively (see Appendices, page 193). The ASHP statement defines the mission of the pharmacist as providing pharmaceutical care, which is "...the direct, responsible provision of medication-related care for the purpose of achieving definite outcomes that improve a patient's quality of life."[3]

The APhA Principles[4] spell out five characteristics of pharmaceutical care:

1. A professional relationship must be established and maintained.

2. Patient-specific medical information must be collected, organized, recorded, and maintained.

3. Patient-specific medical information must be evaluated and a drug therapy plan developed mutually with the patient.

4. The pharmacist must assure that the patient has all supplies, information, and knowledge necessary to carry out the drug therapy plan.

TABLE 1-2

Definition of Pharmaceutical Care

Hepler and Strand's frequently cited definition of pharmaceutical care, published in a landmark report in 1990:

Pharmaceutical care is the responsible provision of drug therapy for the purpose of achieving definite outcomes that improve a patient's quality of life. These outcomes are:

1. Cure of a disease.

2. Elimination or reduction of a patient's symptomatology.

3. Arresting or slowing of a disease process.

4. Preventing a disease or symptomatology.

Pharmaceutical care involves the process through which a pharmacist cooperates with a patient and other professionals in designing, implementing, and monitoring a therapeutic plan that will produce specific therapeutic outcomes for the patient. This in turn involves three major functions:

1. Identifying potential and actual drug-related problems.

2. Resolving actual drug-related problems.

3. Preventing potential drug-related problems.

Pharmaceutical care is a necessary element of health care, and should be integrated with other elements. Pharmaceutical care is, however, provided for the direct benefit of the patient, and the pharmacist is responsible directly to the patient for the quality of that care. The fundamental relationship in pharmaceutical care is a mutually beneficial exchange in which the patient grants authority to the provider and the provider gives competence and commitment (accepts responsibility) to the patient. The fundamental goals, processes, and relationships of pharmaceutical care exist regardless of practice setting.

Source: Hepler CD, Strand LM. Opportunities and responsibilities in pharmaceutical care. Am J Hosp Pharm. 1990;47:533-43.

5. The pharmacist must review, monitor, and modify the therapeutic plan as necessary and appropriate, in concert with the patient and health care team.

The concepts put forth by Hepler and Strand, APhA, and ASHP are prerequisites to delivering any patient care services in pharmacy. Without adopting these philosophies, a pharmacist's ability to commit the resources and effort to provide quality care is diminished. Without commitment, care becomes the unorganized, sporadic delivery of isolated services to customers who are not engaged with their pharmacist.

The Therapeutic Relationship

A key concept in the delivery of pharmaceutical care is the direct responsibility the pharmacist has to the patient. As he goes beyond the role of being consultative to other health care professionals who are actually providing the care, an integral component of pharmaceutical care is the formation of this therapeutic relationship. Patients need to be actively involved in their health care, and it is essential that they develop a trusting and collaborative relationship with health care providers. The pharmacist forms a covenant with the patient: a promise to do whatever is necessary to make sure the patient achieves positive outcomes from drug therapy.

A pharmacist's contributions to this professional relationship include holding the patient's welfare paramount, maintaining an appropriate attitude of caring for the patient's welfare, and using professional knowledge and skills on the patient's behalf. The patient's responsibilities include supplying personal information, expressing preferences, and participating in the development of the care plan. The relationship is facilitated by effective communication, comprehensive data collection, and emphasis on the patient's current and future well-being. (For more information on the therapeutic relationship, see Chapter 3.)

Easier Said than Done

Discussing definitions of pharmaceutical care and how to develop a relationship with patients is much easier than doing it. What does pharmaceutical care look like when it is implemented in practice? It is not just consultation booths, pharmacists' offices, technicians, new computer systems, or detailed patient charts, although all of these may be used and

A key concept in the delivery of pharmaceutical care is the direct responsibility the pharmacist has to the patient.

may be necessary to deliver care. And it is not only about running laboratory tests, performing pharmacokinetic calculations, answering drug information questions, or giving pharmacotherapy consults to physicians, although these are all activities that might occur while providing care. Pharmaceutical care is a philosophy, not forms and fixtures. At the heart it means caring about the patient, and as a health care professional spending the time and effort needed to help another human being.

Pharmacists are providing more varied services than ever before, and this means they must truly get to know their patients. The pharmacist must understand the patients' medications and the status of patients' medical problems, and also find out not only all the medications patients take, but how they take them and how they feel about taking them. In this process they learn more about patients' health care beliefs, including their view of the health care role of the pharmacist. Quality care cannot be provided with only a superficial understanding of the patient.

Pharmaceutical care is a philosophy, not forms or fixtures. At the heart it means caring about the patient.

The pharmacist collects and evaluates information about patients and determines what, if any, problems exist in their current therapeutic regimens. She does this by applying unique knowledge regarding the optimal use of medication to the patient's circumstance. If problems are identified, she seeks a solution, formulates a plan to correct the problem, and puts that plan into effect to help the patient. To do this successfully, the pharmacist needs to apply skills and knowledge beyond that required for traditional dispensing-oriented pharmacy practice.

As the pharmacist spends time talking with a patient to make sure he really understands how to use his dosage form, places a call to the physician to discuss the appropriateness of a drug or dosage, or works with the patient's care providers to develop a system to assure that he actually receives the agreed-upon medication regimen, she is using her skills in practice. As she follows up with her patients the pharmacist seeks to answer questions such as: Did the medicines dispensed actually help the patient? Is his condition resolved or as well controlled as possible? Have the therapy goals that were set been attained? Is the medication regimen causing new problems? Providing pharmaceutical care means that, at the end of the day, pharmacists measure their success by how many people they have helped, not by how many prescriptions they have filled.

A Response to Problems in the System

The current health care system is fraught with problems of quality and safety. The Institute of Medicine report *To Err is Human: Building a Safer Health System*[5] brought the issue of safety in the health care system clearly into public view. It noted that deficiencies in the current drug distribution and medication use systems contribute to more than 44,000 Americans dying per year, with medication errors contributing 7,000 deaths to this number. Two percent of those admitted to a hospital experience a preventable adverse drug event, and each event results in $4,700 additional cost to the health care system.

The recently released IOM report, *Preventing Medication Errors,*[6] expands on the discussion of medication errors, an important safety issue in our health care system. It estimates that 1.5 million preventable adverse drug effects occur each year in the United States. (This number does not include failures to adequately prescribe therapy to prevent or treat medical conditions.) This report further estimates that at least a quarter of these harmful adverse drug effects are preventable.

A significant body of literature speaks to the negative outcomes of drug therapy in individual patients or groups of patients. Manasse[7] reviewed the causes behind the adverse consequences of medication use (his term is "drug misadventuring") and found that adverse drug reaction rates varied widely (0.66% to 50.6%). This and other reports[6,8,9] find that the observed percentage of hospitalizations due to adverse drug reactions also seems to vary widely. Manasse concluded, perhaps conservatively, that up to 10% on average of all hospital admissions might be caused by drug misadventures. Many adverse drug reactions are not recognized as such because patients and providers may tolerate or ignore drug effects, assuming they are part of the condition under treatment or are related to some other disease.

Many adverse outcomes of drug therapy are not identified simply because no one bothered to look for them. Elderly patients may be especially at risk. While there is controversy regarding a link between an increased number of adverse drug reactions and increased age,[10,11] a relationship has been recognized between adverse drug reactions and an increased number of medications.[10] As the population continues to age, problems associated with adverse effects of medications will continue to cause harm to patients unless the current system changes.

Providing pharmaceutical care means that, at the end of the day, pharmacists measure their success by how many people they have helped, not by how many prescriptions they have filled.

Noncompliance (sometimes called nonadherence) with prescribed therapies is another major contributor to drug-related hospitalizations and an important cause of drug-related morbidity and mortality. A meta-analysis by Sullivan et al.[12] found noncompliance to be responsible for 5.3% of hospital admissions. A study of 315 elderly patients admitted to hospitals found that 11.4% of admissions were due to noncompliance, with 32.7% of the patients reporting a history of noncompliance in the previous year.[13] Slightly over half of this nonadherence to prescribed therapy was intentional.

Medication errors and noncompliance are also a problem in patients who have recently been discharged from the hospital. Omori et al.[14] found that 32% of patients were taking a wrong drug and 18% were taking a wrong dose one month after hospital discharge. In this study, a higher number of errors was associated with patients being on more medications at discharge or having more medication changes during hospitalization. Other studies have found that elderly patients on a lower than average number of medications when admitted are at risk of being discharged with a greater number of medications than the average patient.[15] And a study of the elderly found that 43% of patients were unable to adhere to the prescribed regimen for one or more of their prescriptions, and that more than 70% of these intentionally did not adhere.[16]

Patients' Needs Will Expand

The growth of the nonprescription drug market and the continuing conversion of prescription drugs to nonprescription status suggest that patients' need for assistance with self-care will also continue to grow. Patients' burgeoning acceptance and use of alternative therapies, including herbal medicine, vitamins, and homeopathy, is another indication that patients are seeking more from the health care system. A 2002 survey of over 30,000 adults found that 35% had used complementary or alternative medicine in the prior 12 months (excluding prayer and megavitamins). [17]

Nonprescription medications are among the most widely used therapies. Every week more than 40% of people in the United States take a vitamin/mineral product, and 14% take an herbal/supplement.[18] Another survey found that 38% of patients served by a health maintenance organization (HMO) reported using an herbal remedy in the past 12 months.[19] People seem to be increasingly comfortable engaging in self-care.[20] As the most readily accessible health care providers, pharmacists can address the need for assistance with these therapies.

Data on inappropriate prescribing also support the need for change. Willcox et al.[21] reported that 23.5% of an ambulatory elderly population received one or more drugs from a list of 20 considered inappropriate for the elderly. Gonzales et al.[22] found that inappropriate use of antibiotics for conditions in which antibiotics offer little or no benefit accounted for 21% of all antibiotics prescribed to adults.

Findings in these studies present opportunities for pharmacy; if these problems were eliminated or diminished there could be significant positive impact on health care outcomes and costs. Some of these drug therapy problems could be addressed by pharmacists in the course of providing services. Rupp et al.[23] reported that 2.6% of new prescriptions presented at a community pharmacy had errors that required active pharmacist intervention. Approximately 80% of these were prescription-based errors and omissions (incomplete or vague information regarding the drug, strength, or directions). Christensen et al.[24] found that approximately 4% of prescriptions presented to an outpatient HMO contained problems, most commonly drug interactions and drug underuse. Several authors have reported much higher rates of problem identification in patient groups studied over time.[25, 26] This represents the tip of the iceberg when it comes to problems that can be identified in the community pharmacy setting by pharmacists embracing a more active role.

Lowering Costs, Improving Outcomes

Johnson and Bootman[27] in 1995 estimated the annual cost of medication-related morbidity and mortality for the ambulatory population at $76.6 billion, noting that it matches nearly dollar for dollar the amount spent on prescription medications. According to their calculations, the cost could range from $30.1 billion to $136.8 billion, depending on the assumptions used in their model. They also estimated that because of treatment failures or new medical problems developing during therapy, more than 40% of patients would not obtain an optimal outcome of drug therapy under current conditions. In a later report, Johnson and Bootman estimated that 59.6% of the $76.6 billion could be avoided if pharmacists intervened to address drug-related problems.[28] These estimates of drug-related morbidity and mortality were updated in 2000 and at that point were thought to total $177.4 billion.[29]

The literature shows that pharmacists can have an impact on both costs and patient outcomes, and studies are ongoing. In a study from the 1970s, pharmacists in six community pharmacies helped improve compliance and degree of blood pressure control in a hypertensive population study.[30] More recent studies in outpatient clinics of a university health center and a veterans' medical center showed that pharmacists' efforts had a positive effect on blood pressure control[31] and lipids.[32] Ernst et al.[33] described the first year of a pharmacist-provided influenza vaccination program and noted that the pharmacist, who administered 343 doses of vaccine, contributed to an increase in immunization rates over the previous year.

Currie et al.[25] found that the number of drug-related problems identified in a single pharmacy was substantially higher in a population provided pharmaceutical care than in a control group offered traditional pharmacy services. In the pharmaceutical care versus control group, the odds of detecting drug-related problems were 7.5 to 1; the odds of taking action to resolve them were 8.1 to 1. More than 57 drug-related problems per 100 patients were found in the pharmaceutical care group versus three drug-related problems per 100 patients in the control group.

Project ImPACT: Hyperlipidemia showed the ability of pharmacists from across the country to have positive effects on patients' total and LDL cholesterol in a long-term study.[34] Pharmacists in the Asheville Project were able to improve clinical outcome measures of patients with asthma while decreasing overall treatment costs.[35] In a similar pharmaceutical case management project at a self-insured employer's worksite, pharmacists had a positive effect on patients' blood pressure and low-density lipoprotein cholesterol.[36] Expanded care provision by pharmacists in a state-wide Medicaid program resulted in a decrease in use of high-risk medications and an improvement in medication appropriateness.[37]

A recent study found that pharmacists providing individualized medication education, medication dispensing in special adherence packaging, and routine follow-ups increased adherence from 61% to over 96% in an elderly population on multiple medications. In addition to improving medication use, study patients also had improvements in their blood pressure and lipid measures which regressed towards baseline after the services were stopped.[38]

Currie et al. and Cipolle et al. noted a difference in the problems that are identified in patients receiving pharmaceutical care versus the problems identified in the process of dispensing in the community pharmacy setting, such as need for additional drug therapy, wrong drug, adverse drug reaction, and unnecessary drug therapy.[25,26]

Problems such as these are not likely to be identified or addressed without additional care being provided by the pharmacist.

Results of pharmacists providing inpatient care also show a positive impact. In the hospital intensive care setting, Leape et al.[39] found that pharmacist participation on rounds at the time medications were ordered decreased preventable adverse drug events by 72%. Kucukarslan et al.[40] found a 78% decrease in preventable adverse drug events with pharmacist rounding on an inpatient internal medicine service. This is consistent with the finding that the provision of essential clinical pharmacy services and increased staffing levels of clinical pharmacists decrease the rate of adverse drug reactions in hospitalized Medicare patients.[41] Pharmacist involvement in medication reconciliation and counseling on discharge from the hospital can also have a positive effect. Schnipper et al.[42] showed that pharmacists could identify and address a number of different drug-related problems by reviewing medication regimens, counseling patients and discussing these problems with the medical team. Patients receiving this type of care had significantly fewer preventable adverse drug effects and significantly fewer emergency department visits and hospital re-admissions than the usual care group.

In addition to describing the problems in the health care system, the IOM[5] recommended the following actions, among others, to improve patient safety:

• Health professions' performance standards and expectations should focus greater attention on patient safety.

• Health professions should, with their health care organization, continually improve patient safety.

• Health care organizations should implement proven medication safety practices.

Pharmacists providing care is consistent with these methods to identify and address drug therapy problems.

The IOM report, *Preventing Medication Errors*, makes a number of recommendations to improve the safety and quality of the medication use process. These are wide ranging and include empowering patients to become active participants in their care; seeking improvements in patient education, patient and provider drug information, patient history and other information systems; and using technology to study systems for the delivery of care.[6] Pharmacists can help address many problems identified in this report.

There are many causes for medication errors, not all pharmacist-related and not all preventable. However, pharmacists who have knowledge of patients' medical conditions and medications will more easily recognize when an inappropriate drug is ordered, no matter what the cause. They would also have a style of practice that would confirm patient knowledge of all regimens, check for appropriate individualized dosing for the patient based on age, weight, drug elimination, etc., and follow up after new medications are added to a patient's regimen. This approach to therapy addresses several common types of medication errors.[43] Care-oriented pharmacists, more likely to have a better global understanding of the patient's current status, are better able to apply knowledge for the benefit of the patient. Additionally, a practice designed to care for patients with fewer interruptions allows a pharmacist to focus on the patient and avoid errors caused by the many distractions common in the distribution process.

Pharmacists clearly have the potential to be part of the solution to the many problems that have been identified in the medication use process in this country.

Pharmacists clearly have the potential to be part of the solution to the many problems that have been identified in the medication use process in this country. Other literature, as well, has suggested the economic benefits [44-50] and other outcomes [28, 51-63] of pharmaceutical care.

Change and Survival

Despite the obvious need for pharmacists to expand their health care role, many are not taking steps to address this need. A national survey of pharmacists found that 56% of their work time was spent on medication dispensing responsibilities, while only 19% and 9% was spent on consultation and drug management responsibilities, respectively (although the pharmacists wanted to spend more time on these activities).[64]

Pharmacists do not always do all they can to protect the public's health.[65-67] In Gallup polls, pharmacists were consistently rated the most trusted professionals, yet they have fallen in the rankings in recent years. Current reimbursement strategies and incentives often cause pharmacists to focus their attention on increasing prescription volume and maximizing efficiency, making it more difficult for them to spend time working with patients. Pressure on the profession by managed care and pharmacy benefit managers continues. The implementation of the Medicare outpatient prescription drug benefit (Part D) has resulted in significant financial and practice-related stress on community pharmacists. Although Medicare Part D may afford new opportunities to establish professional roles with patients through the provision of Medication Therapy Management Services (MTMS), the ultimate effect is not yet realized.

Although the shift to pharmaceutical care is primarily about helping patients and addressing unmet needs, it is also about the survival of a longstanding profession. Leslie Benet conveyed the stark and uncomfortable scenario toward which pharmacy may be headed in an address to the American Association of Colleges of Pharmacy (AACP) in 1994.[68] If the trend of ever more prescriptions being filled by mail-order pharmacy (which technology is making faster and more efficient) continues, the need for pharmacists will diminish. Only 29,200 pharmacists—one-sixth of the nation's then 170,000 total—would be needed if all prescriptions were eventually handled by mail order. If, however, we move instead to a pharmacist-managed medication review similar to that in a managed care facility, we will need 550,000 pharmacists, or about three times the number at the time, to manage the country's medication needs. As Benet points out, the pharmacy profession can either rally to focus on important health care needs or it can risk becoming virtually extinct.

*Professional
pharmacy groups
and schools
and colleges of
pharmacy have
recognized that
pharmaceutical care
is no passing trend:
it's the future of
pharmacy.*

Professional pharmacy groups and schools and colleges of pharmacy have recognized that pharmaceutical care is no passing trend: it's the future of pharmacy. Increased resources are being dedicated to the effort.[69-72] AACP reaffirmed its position that the mission of pharmacy practice is to deliver pharmaceutical care.[73] AACP also recommended accelerating the pace of reforming college curricula to prepare graduates to provide pharmaceutical care.[74-75] In 2004 the Joint Commission of Pharmacy Practitioners envisioned pharmacists as being responsible for the rational use of medications and accountable for medication use outcomes.[76] The newly published Accreditation Council for Pharmacy Education Standards continue to stress the development of clinically competent pharmacy graduates able to provide pharmaceutical care to patients.[77]

Adapting to change is a necessary part of survival,[78] and change is occurring quickly in the health care system. New drugs, new providers, new professional roles, and new public policy directions reposition the role and the need for pharmacy. While there is comfort in maintaining current practice philosophies and processes, pharmacists cannot ignore the realities of the changing climate. Pharmacy needs to adapt and dedicate substantial resources into transforming to a patient-oriented profession if it is to remain a vital part of the health care environment.

The status quo of our medication use system is no longer acceptable. Over the last several years numerous reports have echoed the call for major reform. The profession of pharmacy must work within itself and with other professions to develop safer and less costly methods to deliver care. Patients need and want pharmacists' help. By committing to a new form of practice and taking immediate steps, they can make pharmaceutical care a reality. For individual practitioners and students still in training, this book should provide solid tips and guidelines for launching a successful pharmaceutical care practice.

Self Assessment Questions

1.1 Review the four patient situations described at the beginning of this chapter. For each one, consider:

- What is the patient's current problem?

- How can the pharmacist assist each of these patients?

- What could the pharmacist have done to prevent the problem from occurring?

1.2 Why is it important to have support systems in place for pharmacists?

1.3 Paraphrase the definition of pharmaceutical care.

1.4 From a societal perspective, why should pharmaceutical care be provided to patients?

1.5 Medication errors are only a part of what is addressed in the provision of pharmaceutical care to patients. What are other important aspects of this type of care?

1.6 List some factors in the health care system that affect the practice of pharmacy and would be positively impacted if pharmacists had a more active role in the delivery of patient care.

Reflection Question

Think about a pharmacy practice you have seen or have worked in. Do patients have all their medication-related health care needs addressed? Are pharmacists actively seeking out patients' drug therapy problems? What opportunities to deliver improved care are left unmet?

References

1. Cipolle RJ. Drugs Don't have Doses—People have Doses! A clinical educator's philosophy. *Drug Intell Clin Pharm.* 1986;20:881-2.

2. Hepler CD, Strand LM. Opportunities and responsibilities in pharmaceutical care. *Am J Hosp Pharm.* 1990;47:533-43.

3. American Society of Hospital Pharmacists. ASHP statement on pharmaceutical care. *Am J Hosp Pharm.* 1993;50:1720-3.

4. *Principles of Practice for Pharmaceutical Care.* Washington, DC: American Pharmaceutical Association; 1995.

5. Kohn LT, Corrigan JM, Donaldson, MS, eds. Committee on Quality of Health Care in America, Institute of Medicine. *To Err is Human: Building a Safer Health System.* Washington, D.C.:National Academy Press; 2000.

6. Aspden P, Wolcott J, Bootman JL, et al., eds. Committee on Identifying and Preventing Medication Errors. *Preventing Medication Errors: Quality Chasm Series.* Washington, D.C.: National Academy Press; 2006. Executive Summary available at http://newton.nap.edu/execsumm_pdf/11623. Accessed August 30, 2006.

7. Manasse HR. Medication use in an imperfect world: drug misadventuring as an issue of public policy, Part 1. *Am J Hosp Pharm.* 1989;46:929-44.

8. McKenney JM, Harrison WL. Drug-related hospital admissions. *Am J Hosp Pharm.* 1976;33:792-5.

9. Caranasos GJ, Steward RB, Cluff LE. Drug-induced illness leading to hospitalization. *JAMA.* 1974;228:713-7.

10. Gurwitz JH, Avorn J. The ambiguous relation between aging and adverse drug reactions. *Ann Intern Med.* 1991;114:956-66.

11. Nolan L, O'Malley K. Prescribing for the elderly: Part I, sensitivity of the elderly to adverse drug reactions. *J Am Geriatr Soc.* 1988;36:142-9.

12. Sullivan SD, Kreling DH, Hazlet TK. Noncompliance with medication regimens and subsequent hospitalization: a literature analysis and cost of hospitalization estimate. *J Res Pharm Econ.* 1990;2:19-33.

13. Col N, Fanale JF, Kronholm P. The role of medication noncompliance and adverse drug reactions in hospitalizations of the elderly. *Arch Intern Med.* 1990;150:841-5.

14. Omori DM, Potyk RP, Kroenke K. The adverse effects of hospitalization on drug regimens. *Arch Intern Med.* 1991;151:1562-4.

15. Beers MH, Dang J, Hasegawa J, et al. Influence of hospitalization on drug therapy in the elderly. *J Am Geriatr Soc.* 1989;37:679-83.

16. Cooper JK, Love DW, Raffoul PR. Intentional prescription nonadherence (noncompliance) by the elderly. *J Am Geriatr Soc*. 1982;30:329-33.

17. Barnes P, Powell-Griner E, McFann K, et al. *CDC Advance Data Report #343*: Complementary and Alternative Medicine Use Among Adults: United States, 2002. May 27, 2004.

18. Kaufman DW, Kelly JP, Rosenberg L, et al. Recent patterns of medication use in the ambulatory adult population of the United States: The Slone Survey. *JAMA*. 2002;287:337-44.

19. Bennett J, Brown CM. Use of herbal remedies by patients in a health maintenance organization. *J Am Pharm Assoc*. 2000;40:353-8.

20. Murphy JC. Americans make choices about self-care. *Am J Health Syst Pharm*. 2001;58:1494-9.

21. Willcox SM, Himmelstein DU, Woolhandler S. Inappropriate drug prescribing for the community-dwelling elderly. *JAMA*. 1994;272:292-6.

22. Gonzales R, Steiner JF, Sande MA. Antibiotic prescribing for adults with colds, upper respiratory tract infections, and bronchitis by ambulatory care physicians. *JAMA*. 1997;278:901-4.

23. Rupp MT, Schondelmeyer SW, Wilson GT, et al. Documenting prescribing errors and pharmacist interventions in community pharmacy practice. *Am Pharm*. 1988;NS28(9):30-7.

24. Christensen DB, Campbell WH, Madsen S, et al. Documenting outpatient problem intervention activities of pharmacists in an HMO. *Med Care*. 1981;19:104-16.

25. Currie JD, Chrischilles EA, Kuehl AK, et al. Effect of a training program on community pharmacists' detection of and intervention in drug-related problems. *J Am Pharm Assoc*. 1997;NS37:182-91.

26. Cipolle RJ, Strand LM, Morley PC. *Pharmaceutical Care Practice*. New York: McGraw-Hill; 1998:219-22.

27. Johnson JA, Bootman JL. Drug-related morbidity and mortality: a cost-of-illness model. *Arch Intern Med*. 1995;155:1949-56.

28. Johnson JA, Bootman JL. Drug-related morbidity and mortality and the economic impact of pharmaceutical care. *Am J Health Syst Pharm*. 1997;54:554-8.

29. Ernst FR, Grizzle AJ. Drug-related morbidity and mortality: updating the cost-of-illness model. *J Am Pharm Assoc*. 2001;41:192-9.

30. McKenney JM, Brown ED, Necsary R, et al. Effect of pharmacist drug monitoring and patient education on hypertensive patients. *Contemp Pharm Pract*. 1978;1(2):50-6.

31. Erickson SR, Slaughter R, Halapy H. Pharmacists' ability to influence outcomes of hypertension therapy. *Pharmacotherapy*. 1997;17:140-7.

32. Konzem SL, Gray DR, Kashyap ML. Effect of pharmaceutical care on optimum colestipol treatment of elderly hypercholesterolemic veterans. *Pharmacotherapy*. 1997;17:576-83.

33. Ernst ME, Chalstrom CV, Currie JD, et al. Implementation of a community pharmacy-based influenza vaccination program. *J Am Pharm Assoc.* 1997;NS37:570-80.

34. Bluml BM, McKenney JM, Cziraky MJ. Pharmaceutical care services and results in Project ImPACT: Hyperlipidemia. *J Am Pharm Assoc.* 2000;40:157-65.

35. Bunting BA, Cranor CW. The Asheville Project: Long-Term Clinical, Humanistic, and Economic Outcomes of a Community-Based Medication Therapy Management Program for Asthma. *J Am Pharm Assoc.* 2006;46:133-47.

36. John EJ, Vavra T, Farris KB, et al. Workplace-Based Cardiovascular Risk Management by Community Pharmacists: Impact on Blood Pressure and Lipid Level. *Pharmacotherapy.* 2006;26(10):1511-17.

37. Chrischilles EA, Carter BL, Lund BC, et al. Evaluation of the Iowa Medicaid Pharmaceutical Case Management Program. *J Am Pharm Assoc.* 2004;44:337-49.

38. Lee JK, Grace KA, Taylor AJ. Effect of a pharmacy care program on medication adherence and persistence, blood pressure, and low-density lipoprotein cholesterol; A randomized controlled trial. *JAMA.* 2006;296:2563-71.

39. Leape LL, Cullen DJ, Clapp MD, et al. Pharmacist participation on physician rounds and adverse drug events in the intensive care unit. *JAMA.* 1999;282(3):267-70.

40. Kucukarslan SN, Peters M, Mlynarek M, et al. Pharmacists on rounding teams reduce preventable adverse drug events in hospital general medicine units. *Arch Intern Med.* 2003;163:2014–8.

41. Bond CA, Raehl CL. Clinical Pharmacy Services, Pharmacy Staffing and Adverse Drug Reactions in United States Hospitals. *Pharmacotherapy.* 2006;26(6):735-47.

42. Schnipper JL, Kirwin JL, Cotugno MC, et al. Role of pharmacist counseling in preventing adverse drug events after hospitalization. *Arch Intern Med.* 2006;166(5):565-71.

43. Cohen MR, ed. *Medication Errors.* Washington, DC: American Pharmaceutical Association; 1999:1.1-1.8.

44. Hatoum HT, Catizone C, Hutchinson RA, et al. An eleven-year review of the pharmacy literature: documentation of the value and acceptance of clinical pharmacy. *Drug Intell Clin Pharm.* 1986;20:33-41.

45. Willett MS, Bertch KE, Rich DS, et al. Prospectus on the economic value of clinical pharmacy services. *Pharmacotherapy.* 1989;9:45-56.

46. Schumock GT, Meek PD, Ploetz PA, et al. Economic evaluation of clinical pharmacy services 1988-1995. *Pharmacotherapy.* 1996;16:1188-208.

47. Dobie RL, Rascati KL. Documenting the value of pharmacist interventions. *Am Pharm.* 1994;NS34:50-4.

48. Rupp MT. Value of community pharmacists' interventions to correct prescribing errors. *Ann Pharmacother.* 1992;26:1580-4.

49. Harrison DL, Bootman JL, Cox ER. Cost-effectiveness of consultant pharmacists in managing drug-related morbidity and mortality at nursing facilities. *Am J Health Syst Pharm.* 1998; 55:1588-94.

50. Schumock GT, Melissa G. Butler MG, Meek PD, et al. Evidence of the Economic Benefit of Clinical Pharmacy Services: 1996–2000. *Pharmacotherapy.* 2003;23(1):113-32.

51. Martin S. Pharmaceutical care made easy. *Am Pharm.* 1994;NS34(3):61-4.

52. Meade V. Pharmaceutical care in a changing health care system. *Am Pharm.* 1994;NS34(8):43-6.

53. Meade V. Adapting to providing pharmaceutical care. *Am Pharm.* 1994; NS34(10):37-42.

54. Meade V. Pharmacist in Richmond launches pharmaceutical care program. *Am Pharm.* 1994;NS34(11):43-5.

55. Meade V. Helping pharmacists provide disease-based pharmaceutical care. *Am Pharm.* 1995;NS35(3):45-8.

56. Bloom MZ. Simple changes reap big rewards. *Am Pharm.* 1995;NS35(8):18-9.

57. Tomechko MA, Strand LM, Morley PC, et al. Q and A from the pharmaceutical care project in Minnesota. *Am Pharm.* 1995;NS35(4):30-9.

58. Grainger-Rousseau TJ, Miralles MA, Hepler CD, et al. Therapeutic outcomes monitoring: application of pharmaceutical care guidelines to community pharmacy. *J Am Pharm Assoc.* 1997;NS37(6):647-61.

59. Nola KM, Gourley DR, Portner TS, et al. Clinical and humanistic outcomes of a lipid management program in the community pharmacy setting. *J Am Pharm Assoc.* 2000;40:166-73.

60. Berringer R, Shibley MCH, Cary CC, et al. Outcomes of a community pharmacy-based diabetes monitoring program. *J Am Pharm Assoc.* 1999;39:791-7.

61. Gourley DR, Gourley GA, Solomon DK, et al. Part 1. Development, implementation, and evaluation of a multicenter pharmaceutical care outcomes study. *J Am Pharm Assoc.* 1998;38:567-73.

62. Solomon DK, Portner TS, Bass GE, et al. Part 2. Clinical and economic outcomes in the hypertension and COPD arms of a multicenter outcomes study. *J Am Pharm Assoc.* 1998;38:574-85.

63. Gourley GA, Portner TS, Gourley DR, et al. Part 3. Humanistic outcomes in the hypertension and COPD arms of a multicenter outcomes study. *J Am Pharm Assoc.* 1998;38:586-97.

64. Schommer JC, Pedersen CA, Doucette WR, et al. Community pharmacists' work activities in the United States during 2000. *J Am Pharm Assoc.* 2002;42:399-406.

65. Headden S, Lenzy T, Kostyu P, et al. Danger at the drugstore. *US News & World Report.* August 25, 1996:46-53.

66. Headden S. The big pill push. *US News & World Report.* September 1, 1997:67-75.

67. Zimmerman A, Armstrong D. Use of pharmacies by drug makers to push pills raises privacy issues. *Wall Street Journal Online*. May 1, 2002. Available at: http://online.wsj.com/article_email/ 0,,SB1020199130825221360,00.html. Accessed May 1, 2002.

68. Benet LZ. Pharmacy education in an era of health care reform. *Am J Pharm Educ*. 1994;58:399-401.

69. Currie JD, McDonough RP, Hagel HP, et al. College of Pharmacy faculty time spent developing pharmaceutical care practice sites [abstract]. *Pharmacotherapy*. 1996;16:141.

70. Rovers J, Hagel H, McDonough R, et al. Impact on college faculty of implementing pharmaceutical care in community pharmacies [abstract]. *Pharmacotherapy*. 1996;16:140.

71. Hagel H. Expanding clinical practice to community pharmacy settings [abstract]. *Pharmacotherapy*. 1996;16:140.

72. Kennedy DT, Ruffin DM, Goode JR, et al. The role of academia in community-based pharmaceutical care. *Pharmacotherapy*. 1997;17(6):1352-6.

73. Commission to Implement Change in Pharmaceutical Education. *Maintaining our commitment to change*. American Association of Colleges of Pharmacy. Alexandria, VA: January 1997.

74. Commission to Implement Change in Pharmaceutical Education. Background Paper I: What is the mission of pharmaceutical education? *Am J Pharm Educ*. 1993;57:374-6.

75. Commission to Implement Change in Pharmaceutical Education. Background Paper II: Entry level, curricular outcomes, curricular content and educational process. *Am J Pharm Educ*. 1993;57:377-85.

76. JCPP Writing Team. *JCPP Future Vision of Pharmacy Practice*. Adopted November 10, 2004. Available at: http://www.aacp.org/Docs/ MainNavigation/Resources/6725_JCPPFutureVisionofPharmacyPracticeFINAL.pdf. Accessed August 23, 2006.

77. Accreditation Council for Pharmacy Education. *Accreditation Standards and Guidelines for the Professional Program in Pharmacy Leading to the Doctor of Pharmacy Degree*. Adopted January 15, 2006. Available at: http://www.acpe-accredit.org/deans/standards.asp. Accessed August 23, 2006.

78. Handy C. *The Age of Paradox*. Boston: Harvard Business School Press; 1994:50-67.

Notes

Identifying Drug Therapy Problems

2

John P. Rovers

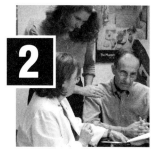

This is the first of four chapters about the process of practicing pharmaceutical care and how to care for patients. Simply put, the practice of pharmaceutical care is the deliberate act of finding and resolving drug therapy problems.

The pharmacy literature first described drug therapy problems over 10 years ago,[1] and they provide a well-defined and defensible structure for the scope of pharmacy practice. Since pharmacy is changing so rapidly, defining this scope is necessary to ensure that pharmacists work only within their areas of competency and to convince payers that pharmacists are seeking to be paid only for specific, definable, cognitive tasks that they are best equipped to perform.

There are only seven drug therapy problems, outlined in Table 2-1, so it is easy to tell when you are practicing pharmaceutical care.

Drug therapy problems are not dispensing errors or other accidental variations from what the prescriber intended the patient to receive. Such errors and variations are simply mistakes.

TABLE 2-1

The Seven Drug Therapy Problems

The seven drug therapy problems that pharmaceutical care addresses are:

- Unnecessary drug therapy.
- Wrong drug (sometimes called ineffective drug).
- Dosage too low.
- Adverse drug reaction.
- Dosage too high.
- Inappropriate compliance (sometimes called adherence).
- Needs additional drug therapy.

In this chapter, the following concepts are reviewed:

- Identifying and preventing or resolving drug therapy problems.

- The etiology of drug therapy problems.

- Five needs for drug therapy and seven drug therapy problems that can result.

- The causes for each drug therapy problem.

- Communicating with patients and other clinicians about drug therapy problems.

- The Pharmaceutical Care Cycle.

- How drug therapy problems are consistent with cognitive services like disease state management, medication reconciliation, medication therapy management services, and others.

The next chapters will cover what drug therapy problems are, how to gather the necessary information to find them, how to identify and resolve them, and how to document them. Finding and fixing drug therapy problems is at the heart of the highest quality patient care. These activities are also consistent with the various disease management and screening programs currently offered in many innovative pharmacies. No matter what style of pharmacy practice pharmacists ultimately embrace, drug therapy problems are relevant.

The Pharmaceutical Care Cycle

So how does a pharmaceutical care practice differ from a traditional one that already includes lots of patient counseling and other clinical activities? And how does it differ from the clinical pharmacy that has been practiced in hospitals for several decades? In community pharmacies, perhaps the biggest difference is that pharmaceutical care is cyclical while traditional patient care is episodic. To use an analogy, traditional care is a snapshot of the patient, rather than a video that would give the pharmacist a perspective on everything going on with the patient's health.

Drug therapy problems are not dispensing errors or other accidental variations from what the prescriber intended the patient to receive. Such errors and variations are simply mistakes.

In a traditional patient-oriented practice, the pharmacist provides education and other services that are intended to fix an immediate problem or complaint. There is rarely any organized attempt to find out if the problem has been solved or if new problems have arisen.

Pharmacy students can usually successfully describe an example of a pharmacist–patient interaction from their practice. But they can rarely discuss whether the patient's problem was resolved or if further action was required. Clearly, traditional patient care, no matter how skillfully provided, does not permit pharmacists to assess if they helped their patients, made things worse, or had no impact at all.

Clinical pharmacy has always had excellent patient care as its goal, but the client was typically the physician or nurse. A pharmacist on rounds or performing therapeutic drug monitoring would usually discuss problems or patient care issues with them, but not directly with the patient. In a pharmaceutical care practice, talking with the patient is a vital component to uncovering more and different drug therapy problems.

The practice of pharmaceutical care involves an ongoing series of steps, as illustrated in the diagram of the Pharmaceutical Care Cycle (Figure 2-1). Once a pharmacist finds a patient is eligible to receive pharmaceutical care, the entry point to the cycle is identifying a drug therapy problem.

Few pharmacists have the time, skills or resources to offer pharmaceutical care to every patient who may need it. Instead, they must use a qualifying process to determine to which patients they will offer these services. This qualifying process can be as informal as asking patients getting refill prescriptions if they have any questions or concerns. Patients who answer yes may be offered additional services. Pharmacists offering disease state management programs will find it useful to develop some additional screening questions to determine if patients require help with other health conditions.

In the hospital, all patients admitted via the emergency room or patients on specific medical or surgical floors may qualify. Patients on certain medications (e.g., non-formulary or high risk medications or those drugs targeted for intravenous to oral conversion) may also automatically qualify to receive pharmaceutical care.

As Medication Therapy Management Services (MTMS) develop, it is likely that each insurance company offering Medicare Part D coverage will develop criteria for which patients are eligible to receive MTMS. Thus, pharmacists will need to develop some screening questions for their Medicare Part D patients to see if they qualify for more advanced services. They will also want to check with each insurance plan they accept and determine its specific criteria to assure that the screening questions are appropriate.

Identifying Drug Therapy Problems

The practice of pharmaceutical care is the deliberate act of finding and resolving drug therapy problems.

FIGURE 2-1

The Pharmaceutical Care Cycle

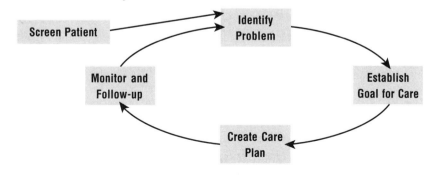

Source: Rovers J. Des Moines, IA: Drake University College of Pharmacy. Used with permission.

To further amplify the cycle shown in Figure 2-1, the pharmacist starts by asking himself if the patient has a drug therapy problem—the "identify problem" step. If the answer is yes, the pharmacist should determine what to do and set a therapeutic goal for the patient. After that, he must decide how best to achieve the goal. He develops and implements a care plan. After the plan is in place, he performs adequate patient follow-up and monitoring to determine if the therapeutic goal has been achieved.

Follow-up can be done formally (by appointment) in community pharmacies or outpatient clinics, or informally when patients come back to the pharmacy for a medication refill or to purchase nonprescription medications. If follow-up is done informally the pharmacist will need to place some kind of alert or reminder in the patient's computer record to prompt her to ask the patient some follow-up questions.

The Pharmaceutical Care Cycle never stops. At each follow-up visit, the pharmacist will ask a few screening questions to determine if the problem has been resolved or if a new problem has arisen. If the patient is stable and has no new problems, nothing further is done until the next scheduled follow-up. If the goal has not been achieved, or if the patient subsequently develops a new drug therapy problem, the Pharmaceutical Care Cycle begins again. Each time the pharmacist detects a drug therapy problem, it is a cue for him to act.

Drug Therapy Problems, Not Medical Problems

It is important to understand the difference between medical problems and drug therapy problems. A medical problem is a disease state; that is, a problem related to altered physiology resulting in clinical evidence of damage. A drug therapy problem, however, is a problem a patient has that is either caused by or may be treated with a drug. Every time a pharmacist finds a patient with any kind of health care question or problem, she should ask herself if a drug caused it or if a drug will be needed to fix it. If the answer to either question is yes, the patient likely has a drug therapy problem.

Who finds and fixes medical problems? Physicians, nurse practitioners, and physician assistants. And who finds and fixes drug therapy problems? Certainly pharmacists, as well as the providers listed above, all spend some of their time finding and fixing drug therapy problems. But if we define responsibility as getting

A medical problem is a disease state, a problem related to altered physiology resulting in clinical evidence of damage. A drug therapy problem is a problem a patient has that is either caused by or may be treated with a drug.

paid to perform a particular service, there is no one practitioner specifically charged with working on drug therapy problems.

This may change under MTMS. Once pharmacists are paid specifically to manage drug therapy, they will be the health care professionals who are charged with the responsibility of working on drug therapy problems. The specific role pharmacists will play is likely to vary according to the benefits provided under each insurance plan.

Drug therapy problems typically develop out of medical problems. For instance, diabetes mellitus, a disease in which glucose is inadequately metabolized, results in damage to the eyes, kidneys and other organs that contain small blood vessels. Thus, diabetes is a medical problem.

However, patients with diabetes can have a variety of drug therapy problems. A patient who needs insulin but goes untreated has a drug therapy problem because she needs the medication to treat her medical problem. In other words, diabetes is not a drug therapy problem, but the need for drug therapy to treat it is. If the patient is not compliant with her insulin therapy and later develops kidney problems, the kidney disease is a medical problem but the poor compliance is a drug therapy problem.

In practice, such distinctions are essential. While a medical problem is the responsibility of the physician, a pharmacist's practice must be limited only to drug therapy problems. As pharmacists provide pharmaceutical care, they learn to distinguish between the two types of problems and must ensure that they are not inadvertently trying to diagnose medical conditions. They must not allow themselves to be drawn into discussions of diagnostic medicine even when patients ask for their opinions.

Using the standardized taxonomy of the seven drug therapy problems keeps pharmacists focused on matters that are clearly within the scope of their practice. Once a physician or other medical professional has diagnosed a disease state, the pharmacist can address drug therapy problems related to which drug or dose to use. And identifying adverse effects or compliance problems are very much consistent with the practice of pharmacy.

As noted in Tables 2-1 and 2-2, pharmacists use a well defined taxonomy to describe the problems that they find and fix or prevent. But they are the only providers in the system who use this terminology. Imagine the potential confusion that can arise when discussing drug therapy problems with physicians or patients not familiar with the terms. For instance, to other practitioners the phrase "drug therapy problem" can be baffling. How can a drug have a problem? People may even conclude that pharmacy's use of the phrase reflects a lack of patient focus.

It is important for pharmacists to rephrase "drug therapy problems" as "the problem a patient may have with his drug therapy." Although the patient may have the drug therapy problem of "dose too low," when discussing the case with nonpharmacists it may be helpful to discuss the patient's "not responding to the current dose." See Box 2-1 for more information on communication skills needed to discuss drug therapy problems.

Discovering Drug Therapy Problems

When pharmacists evaluate their current practices, it is apparent that they already find and solve drug therapy problems. Each day, pharmacists discover drug interactions and therapeutic duplications, speak to physicians, educate patients, and do what is necessary to solve the problems they uncover. Are such pharmacists practicing pharmaceutical care? The answer lies, in part, in how the average pharmacist currently uncovers drug therapy problems compared to how the pharmaceutical care practitioner completes the process after a drug therapy problem is identified.

Often pharmacists do not find problems so much as problems find pharmacists.

Pharmacists determine that a patient has a problem related to a drug in several ways. Usually something about the dose, dosage interval, or duration of therapy may seem unusual when the pharmacist is filling a prescription. And many drug therapy problems are identified when the drug utilization review module of the pharmacist's dispensing software or the third-party payer's claims computer indicates a possible drug interaction, therapeutic duplication, or compliance problem.

The examples above represent problems with prescriptions, not patients with problems. Also, the pharmacist noticed these issues while routinely filling the prescriptions. Often pharmacists do not find problems so much as problems find pharmacists; their discoveries are not purposeful or organized, but accidental. Actively searching for drug therapy problems requires pharmacists to either gather new data to evaluate, or look at the existing data in a new fashion. These ideas will be explored further in Chapters 3 and 4.

A PRACTICAL GUIDE TO PHARMACEUTICAL CARE: A Clinical Skills Primer

An organized approach is critical to success. A study by Currie et al. on a program that trained pharmacists in detecting drug therapy problems showed that when the problems were identified by the usual methods, pharmacists found an average of three per 100 patients.[2] However, when trained pharmacists looked for drug therapy problems, they found an average of 57.6 problems per 100 patients. Overall pharmacists who used an organized approach were 7.5 times more likely to find a drug therapy problem than pharmacists identifying problems by the usual methods.

Cipolle et al.[3] found the most common drug therapy problem is "needs additional drug therapy" (31%) followed by "dosage too low" (22%) and "adverse drug reaction" and "noncompliance" (both 14%). Most patients had only one drug therapy problem while 8-14% had two. In patients under age 65, diabetes, depression, asthma, and menopause were the medical conditions most often associated with a drug therapy problem. In patients over age 65, arthritis, hypertension, anxiety, and hyperlipidemia were the most common medical conditions associated with drug therapy problems.

These results are similar to those found by Hagel and Rovers.[4] In their study of ambulatory elderly patients, the most common drug therapy problems were "needs additional drug therapy" (46%), "noncompliance" (18%) and "dosage too low" (11%). Patients had an average of three drug therapy problems each and the medications involved were most commonly vitamins/nutritionals (26%), cardiac/fluid (17%), and antilipemics (5%).

In a pharmaceutical care practice, pharmacists look for problems that they would not or could not otherwise identify. The following example is based on an actual patient case.

Neil Poole, who received his degree 3 months ago, is performing a medication reconciliation for Ken Tyler, a 67-year-old man admitted to County Hospital through the emergency room with a probable thrombotic stroke. Ken's family brought his home medications to the hospital, including warfarin 1 mg tablets for atrial fibrillation, esomeprazole 20 mg for gastric reflux, and an albuterol inhaler for occasional mild asthma. Neil is comparing the pill vials from Ken's home medications to those listed on his in-patient nursing medication administration sheet (MAR). Other than a switch to the formulary agent omeprazole, Neil's assessment is that Ken's hospital medications are the correct ones.

How might a more experienced Neil Poole, who has a better understanding of drug therapy problems, handle the same situa-

Not all drug therapy problems can be identified from the prescription, a profile review, and screening software. Pharmaceutical care practitioners make a point of gathering additional information to ensure that the intended outcome of therapy is achieved and that no drug therapy problems occur.

tion? Rather than concluding that Ken's medications were appropriate after comparing pill vials and MAR sheets, Neil speaks to Ken's wife, Pat, and asks how he took his medications at home. Pat replies that Ken has taken warfarin 3 mg to 5 mg tablets once a day for years, always as a single tablet. But last month a new physician's assistant changed Ken's dose to 3 mg and prescribed 1 mg tablets with instructions to take 3 tablets daily.

When Neil compared the date on the vial to the pill count, it became apparent that Ken has only been taking one tablet a day. Pat and Neil assume that Ken was so used to taking warfarin once a day that he did not read the instructions on the new vial. His stroke and hospitalization are a direct result of the drug therapy problem of inadvertent noncompliance.

Neil had the experience to know that not all drug therapy problems can be found using traditional screening techniques, and that communication with patients or their caregivers is vital. Neil found this drug therapy problem because he was trying to. He uncovered information not readily available using only profiles and screening software.

Not all drug therapy problems can be identified from the prescription, a profile review, and screening software. Pharmaceutical care practitioners make a point of gathering additional information to ensure that the intended outcome of therapy is achieved and that no drug therapy problems occur. They learn to look at the existing information differently when doing patient counseling, recommending nonprescription therapy, or filling prescriptions.

TABLE 2-2

Five Steps in the Pharmaceutical Care Process

The five steps in the Pharmaceutical Care Process include:

1. A professional relationship with the patient must be established.

2. Patient-specific medical information must be collected, organized, recorded, and maintained.

3. Patient-specific medical information must be evaluated and a drug therapy plan developed mutually with the patient.

4. The pharmacist must ensure that the patient has all supplies, information, and knowledge necessary to carry out the drug therapy plan.

5. The pharmacist must review, monitor, and modify the therapeutic plan as necessary and appropriate, in concert with the patient and health care team.

So, it would appear that pharmacists who discover problems are partial providers of pharmaceutical care. But without a more formal understanding of what drug therapy problems are and how to find them in a consistent, logical, and organized fashion, pharmacists cannot identify all such problems and provide the level of care their patients require. Until then, pharmacists will discover most drug therapy problems inadvertently.

Beyond Counseling

The APhA *Principles of Practice for Pharmaceutical Care* describes five steps to the pharmaceutical care process (see Table 2-2).[5] As a pharmacist carries out the activities required to perform each of these steps, he is practicing pharmaceutical care.

Drug therapy problems may be identified during steps 2 and 3, since this is where the pharmacist gathers patient-specific data and critically examines the data to determine if problems exist. Implicit in these five steps is the reality that providing pharmaceutical care requires an entire shift of focus for pharmacy practice; instead of focusing on product alone, the pharmacist must accept a new level of responsibility.

In traditional dispensing practices, pharmacists were simply responsible for dispensing prescriptions accurately, as prescribed. In these practices, pharmacists assumed responsibility for ensuring that the right patient got the right quantity of the right medication of the right strength at the right time.

Since 1990, most states have mandated patient counseling for all patients obtaining prescription medications. Using a counseling model of practice, pharmacists assume responsibility for ensuring that patients understand key aspects of the use of medications.

In a pharmaceutical care model of practice, the pharmacist goes far beyond counseling to assume responsibility for all the patient's drug-related needs. These needs are summarized in Table 2-3. An understanding of these patient needs is important because whenever one or more of a patient's drug-related needs are not met, a drug therapy problem develops. So, if pharmaceutical care means finding and fixing drug therapy problems, by definition, pharmacists will have to assume responsibility for ensuring that a patient's drug-related needs are being met.

Problems develop when a patient's drug therapy needs are not fully met. Let's consider the consequences of each of these needs.

In a dispensing model of practice, pharmacists assumed responsibility for ensuring that the right patient got the right quantity of the right medication of the right strength at the right time. Using a counseling model of practice, pharmacists assume responsibility for ensuring that patients understand key aspects of the use of medications. In a pharmaceutical care model of practice, the pharmacist goes far beyond counseling to assume responsibility for all the patient's drug-related needs.

Five Key Drug-Related Needs of Patients

Pharmacists who provide pharmaceutical care must ensure that the following needs are met:

1. Patients need every medication they are taking to have an appropriate indication.

2. Patients need their drug therapy to be effective.

3. Patients need their drug therapy to be safe.

4. Patients need to be able to comply with drug therapy and other aspects of their care plans.

5. Patients need to receive all drug therapies necessary to resolve any untreated indications.

• *Patients need every medication they are taking to have an appropriate indication.*
If a drug does not have an appropriate indication, the drug therapy problem "unnecessary drug therapy" will be identified.

• *Patients need their drug therapy to be effective.*
When a patient's need for medication to be effective is not met, two possible drug therapy problems can arise. They are "wrong drug" and "dosage too low."

• *Patients need their drug therapy to be safe.*
Not meeting a need for medication safety can result in the drug therapy problems of "dosage too high" or "adverse drug reaction."

• *Patients need to be able to comply with drug therapy and other aspects of their care plans.*
If a patient is not compliant with her medication the drug therapy problem of "noncompliance" results.

• *Patients need to receive all drug therapies necessary to resolve any untreated indications.*
Finally, patients need all of their medical indications to be treated by some kind of therapy. When that missing therapy is a drug (as opposed to surgery or dietary therapy, etc.), the drug therapy problem of "needs additional drug therapy" is identified. Some pharmacists who perform significant amounts of patient education interpret this problem to encompass the issue of "needs additional education."

Only after each of these five needs has been evaluated and the pharmacist feels confident that each is being met in the optimal fashion can she conclude that the patient does not have a drug therapy problem. The relationship between patients' needs and drug therapy problems is summarized in Table 2-4.

Next let's consider an example of how needs and drug therapy problems are related.

Catherine VerPlank has been admitted for induction chemotherapy for breast cancer with paclitaxel and cisplatin. She receives prophylaxis for chemotherapy-induced nausea and vomiting with ondansetron 4 mg iv 30 minutes prior to chemotherapy. Catherine suffers significant vomiting after her chemotherapy treatment. Her medication need was for the ondansetron to be effective. Since she vomited, that need was not met.

There are two possible drug therapy problems that explain why. Either ondansetron is the wrong drug for Catherine or the dose she received is too low. Since ondansetron is both indicated and widely considered effective for chemotherapy induced emesis and the usual dose of ondansetron is 8–12 mg, we would conclude that the likely drug therapy problem is dosage too low.

How does a pharmacist evaluate all of these patient needs? For example, how can he determine if the patient has an appropriate indication for all drug therapy when he doesn't know what condition the drug is treating? Clearly, current practice methods do not allow the pharmacist to assess all a patient's needs and practice in a manner fully consistent with pharma-

TABLE 2-4

Problems Resulting from Unmet Drug-Related Needs

Drug-Related Need	Drug Therapy Problem
Appropriate indication	1. Unnecessary drug therapy
Effectiveness	2. Wrong drug
	3. Dosage too low
Safety	4. Adverse drug reaction
	5. Dosage too high
Compliance	6. Inappropriate compliance
Untreated indication	7. Needs additional drug therapy

Source: Tomechko MA, Strand LM, Morley PC, et al. Q and A from the pharmaceutical care project in Minnesota. Am Pharm. 1995;NS35(4):30-9.

ceutical care. To do so, the pharmacist will need to gather a patient-specific history. See Chapter 3 for a complete discussion of how this is accomplished.

Causes of Drug Therapy Problems

Patients only have five drug-related needs. When one of these needs is not met, one of seven drug therapy problems can develop. Similarly, each drug therapy problem has a limited number of causes. As pharmacists gather history, evaluate data, and identify drug therapy problems, they must also determine the cause of each problem.

Identifying the cause of a drug therapy problem is important because it suggests potential therapeutic plans that may be implemented. Once you know why a problem occurred, knowing how to fix it becomes easier. Determining the cause can also prevent the pharmacist from developing a plan that does not ultimately assist the patient.

For example, if the drug therapy problem of inappropriate compliance is identified, most pharmacists react by counseling the patient on the benefits of taking his medication correctly. But counseling will only be effective if the patient does not take his medication because he does not understand or agree with the instructions. If a patient is noncompliant with therapy because he cannot swallow a large tablet, what the patient needs is a different drug or dosage form. Identifying the cause of a problem usually suggests a solution.

Each of the drug therapy problems in Table 2-4 has a limited number of causes, as shown in Table 2-5. The tables illustrate that present methods of problem identification are insufficient. Although the methods commonly used in pharmacies today may allow pharmacists to identify occasional problems with prescriptions, not all problems and causes can be identified without further data. For example, it would be impossible for a pharmacist to determine if additional drug therapy is needed unless he is aware of the patient's current medical conditions. A pharmaceutical care approach to practice is needed to identify a patient who has a problem rather than a problem with a prescription.

Without this approach only a small proportion of drug therapy problems will be discovered and acted upon. And even if a problem is identified, without adequate data it is difficult to determine why the problem occurred. In such a case, there is little the

TABLE 2-5

Causes of Drug Therapy Problems

Drug Therapy Problem	Cause
Unnecessary drug therapy	No medical indication
	Addiction/recreational drug use
	Nondrug therapy more appropriate
	Duplicate therapy
	Treating avoidable adverse reaction
Wrong drug	Dosage form inappropriate
	Contraindication present
	Condition refractory to drug
	Drug not indicated for condition
	More effective drug available
Dosage too low	Wrong dosage
	Frequency inappropriate
	Duration inappropriate
	Incorrect storage
	Incorrect administration
	Drug interaction
Adverse drug reaction	Unsafe drug for patient
	Allergic reaction
	Incorrect administration
	Drug interaction
	Dosage increased or decreased too quickly
	Undesirable effect
Dosage too high	Wrong dose
	Frequency inappropriate
	Duration inappropriate
	Drug interaction
Inappropriate compliance	Drug product not available
	Cannot afford drug product
	Cannot swallow or otherwise administer drug
	Does not understand instructions
	Patient prefers not to take drug
Needs additional drug therapy	Untreated condition
	Synergistic therapy
	Prophylactic therapy

Source: Tomechko MA, Strand LM, Morley PC, et al. Q and A from the pharmaceutical care project in Minnesota. Am Pharm. 1995;NS35(4):30•9.

pharmacist can do other than provide further patient counseling and patient education.

A pharmaceutical care practitioner, however, could determine if the patient is noncompliant because he has had an adverse effect, cannot afford the drug, or simply does not believe that the drug works, for instance. Once the cause is known, the appropriate intervention becomes clear.

Actual and Potential Drug Therapy Problems

Drug therapy problems can be one of two types: actual or potential. An actual problem is one that has already occurred. A potential problem is one that is likely to occur—something the patient is at risk of developing—if the pharmacist does not intervene. When an actual drug therapy problem exists, the pharmacist should take action to resolve it. If there is a potential drug therapy problem, the pharmacist should take the necessary steps to prevent it.

When an actual drug therapy problem exists, the pharmacist should take action to resolve it. If there is a potential drug therapy problem, the pharmacist should take the necessary steps to prevent it.

Is the following problem actual or potential? A pharmacist is counseling a patient about a new amoxicillin prescription and learns that he has a history of immediate hypersensitivity reactions to penicillin. As shown in Table 2-5, this problem would be identified as an adverse drug reaction caused by an allergic reaction. The problem is potential since the patient did not actually suffer an allergic reaction to the new prescription. Even if the patient took the amoxicillin, the problem remains potential unless he develops signs and symptoms of an allergic reaction.

Sometimes the pharmacist cannot be certain about a problem because she does not have enough information to identify it conclusively. Suppose, for example, that after screening a patient's profile, the pharmacist believes him to be noncompliant with his high blood pressure medication. Until she can definitely confirm that he is not taking the medication as directed or that the physician changed the dose, she cannot really determine if this is a drug therapy problem or not. Some pharmacists might identify this as a potential problem.

Some drug therapy problems cannot be determined to be actual or potential without additional information. They can be designated "need more information"; this is a way to indicate that more work must be done to determine if a problem exists. Once the pharmacist has gathered additional patient history, a more definitive identification of the problem can be made and the pharmacist can describe the problem as actual or potential with confidence.

Actual and potential problems can be a sticky issue in the pharmacist–physician relationship. In a typical pharmacy practice, most interventions with prescribers are related to potential problems. Often physicians do not take these problems as seriously as pharmacists do.

One common example is drug–drug interactions. Unless the patient is actually suffering from toxicity or lack of clinical effect because of an interaction, this is a potential drug therapy problem. The pharmacist may inform the physician of the potential

BOX 2-1

Communication Tip: Pay Attention to Word Choice

It's important to pay attention to the words used to define certain problems and causes. Phrases such as "wrong drug" or "duration inappropriate" may be accurate in describing the patient's problem, but they carry a negative connotation. When communicating with a physician about a drug therapy problem, remember that pharmaceutical care is new for the rest of the health care system and can be seen as a potential threat. The people who work in that system may not appreciate a pharmacist's opinion that the "wrong drug" was prescribed.

Some people feel personally criticized when such terms are used, and it's easy to see why. It sounds like you are telling them that they made a mistake and blaming them for the situation.

Sometimes, phrasing a problem as a question may be more socially acceptable. For example, a pharmacist fills a new prescription for amlodipine 10 mg tablets to be taken once daily. Since the dose appears to be high, she confirms with the patient that the drug is for mild hypertension that has just been diagnosed. The patient has never tried other drugs for his blood pressure. The pharmacist contacts the physician's office and informs the nurse that the dosage of amlodipine is "too high." A few minutes later, the nurse calls back, sounding annoyed, and simply confirms that the physician wants a dosage of 10 mg.

Now imagine the same clinical scenario with a few changes. The pharmacist phones the physician's office and tells the nurse that she does not often see initial 10 mg amlodipine dosages and would like to clarify how the dosage was selected so that she may better understand how the physician intends to treat this patient. She also indicates that this knowledge will assist her in helping the patient achieve the outcome the physician intends. Depending on the answer received, this more low-key approach allows the pharmacist to recommend a new dosage that "may have less risk of side effects," or "may be just as effective and may be safer."

In each case the same problem is identified. But in the second situation the problem was communicated in a way that is less likely to be interpreted as negative. A physician who is not placed on the defensive because the drug therapy problem is poorly stated is more likely to be receptive to a pharmacist's suggestions. The implication for pharmacists is essentially this: document the problem fully, but be careful with the wording when presenting it to other health care providers.

problem only to find that he continues with the original therapy. To some physicians, unless the interaction is potentially lethal (such as an interaction involving warfarin), potential problems are exactly that. The consequences must be very severe before these physicians are motivated to act.

The outcome is usually different in pharmacist–physician interactions involving actual drug therapy problems. For example, if a pharmacist discovers that a patient is noncompliant with his expensive cholesterol-lowering agent because he cannot afford it, the physician is typically more motivated to prescribe another medication. The physician knows that unless the problem is fixed, the intended outcome of therapy will not be achieved.

While pharmacists should not conclude that potential drug therapy problems do not require action, before deciding to contact a physician they should consider how severe the consequences of the potential problem could be. The risks of prescribing penicillin to a patient who has had a previous allergic reaction are far different from those of giving ibuprofen to a patient with a history of mild gastric upset from diclofenac. In both cases the pharmacist should still act on the problem, but the latter is less likely to require the physician's intervention.

Most pharmacists already try to eliminate unnecessary phone calls to physicians by setting the threshold of their drug interaction screening software high enough so only clinically relevant interactions are likely to be flagged. As pharmacists develop into full-fledged pharmaceutical care practitioners, they will treat a wider variety of drug therapy problems in a similar manner.

What should a pharmacist do when the physician does not agree with her concern about a possible drug therapy problem? Many pharmacists may stop at that point. The pharmaceutical care practitioner, however, can usually identify another course of action. If the physician refuses to act, it falls to the pharmacist to monitor the patient appropriately and to educate him about what to watch out for and when to call the pharmacist or physician for help. The pharmacist must do so in a way that will not damage the physician–patient relationship or cause the patient to question the physician's judgment or competence.

This approach forces the pharmacist to evaluate drug therapy outcomes, which will improve her clinical judgment and result in a more productive discussion on those occasions when the physician must be contacted. In other words, she will develop a better sense of judgment for when to call a physician and when she can handle a problem on her own.

Finding and resolving drug therapy problems may require a new thought process, but it is similar to the kind of thought process most pharmacists already employ. Pharmacists are already trained to examine prescriptions and identify potential problems; pharmaceutical care takes this process one step further, to the patient. The most challenging aspects of providing pharmaceutical care are learning to focus on the patient, ask the right questions, and develop good investigative and research skills.

Drug Therapy Problems and Other Models of Practice

Practicing pharmaceutical care is widely accepted in the profession of pharmacy, but has not been consistently embraced. Instead, a wide variety of disease management, patient education, vaccination, medication reconciliation, and disease screening programs have emerged over the last 10 to 15 years. There is no doubt that these new programs are useful improvements in pharmacists' ability to care for patients. But in many cases these programs are focused on a single issue. Many of them are also limited to a single pharmacist–patient interaction. As valuable as these new initiatives are, they can be made better by widening their focus to include drug therapy problems.

Disease State Management and Patient Education Programs

Disease state management programs in diabetes, asthma, and hyperlipidemia are popular offerings from pharmacists who seek to expand their practices. Most of these programs include a series of pharmacist–patient meetings that occur over several weeks. Although sessions and programs vary widely, a significant amount of the content of most of them is educational. For example, an asthma program would likely include a session on peak flow monitoring and one in diabetes would discuss sick day diabetes management or home blood glucose monitoring. Such information is not typically covered by physicians or by pharmacists who use traditional patient care models. In such cases, it may be reasonable to interpret the drug therapy problem of "needs additional drug therapy" to include "needs additional education." As patient education programs become more popular, pharmacists will need to explain to patients and payers the scope of the educational services they offer. Using a modified drug therapy problem taxonomy is one way to do that.

Finding and resolving drug therapy problems may require a new thought process, but it is similar to the kind of thought process most pharmacists already employ.

Some disease management programs do require the pharmacist to manage the patient's drug therapy. Although these programs often do not use drug therapy problem terminology, pharmacists working with patients do find and solve problems related to all seven drug therapy problems. Documentation systems could be modified so that pharmacists perform drug therapy problem assessment and resolution as part of the program.

Vaccination Programs

Prior to administering a vaccine, pharmacists must determine if it is indicated in a specific patient. If so, the pharmacist administers the vaccine and resolves the drug therapy problem of "needs additional drug therapy." However, vaccination programs can include a wider assessment of drug therapy problems. The data collection tools and methods used to determine the patient's need for a vaccine could be readily modified to include opportunities to assess all five of a patient's drug therapy needs. An assessment of compliance, safety, and efficacy of the patient's drug therapy in general would transform a relatively simple vaccination program into a high quality patient care service.

Medication Reconciliation

This relatively new concept in pharmacy is typically practiced in health systems settings and has become a recent requirement by the Joint Commission on Accreditation of Healthcare Organizations (JCAHO). Problems and errors with medications have long been common in patients being admitted to or discharged from hospitals. Medication reconciliation pharmacists compare the medication prescribed prior to and during hospitalization. Any discrepancies must be investigated and resolved. Medication reconciliation can also be performed when patients are transferred within the hospital (e.g., into or out of a critical care unit) or discharged.

Ideally, medication reconciliation will also include a pharmacist speaking with the patient and/or caregiver. This allows for an assessment of all the patient's drug therapy needs and subsequent identification of any problems. As discussed earlier in this chapter, screening using only computers and drug lists cannot identify all drug therapy problems. Consequently, medication reconciliation pharmacists who also speak to patients and perform an assessment of drug needs will be able to offer high quality pharmaceutical care.

Disease Screening Programs

With the advent of Clinical Laboratory Improvement Amendments (CLIA)-waived testing, pharmacists have been able to provide a number of low complexity diagnostic screening tests in community pharmacies and elsewhere. The most common examples include screenings for osteoporosis, diabetes, hypertension, and hyperlipidemia. In most cases, these screenings require only a single patient visit. After receiving the patient's written consent, the pharmacist draws blood or otherwise performs the necessary testing and provides the patient with a written copy of the results and an interpretation of what the results mean. Patients whose results are outside the normal range are generally encouraged to discuss them with their physician.

Incorporating concepts of pharmaceutical care and drug therapy problem solving into disease screening programs is more difficult than with some of the other pharmacy practice innovations. Screenings in a single visit that do not include a follow-up are conceptually inconsistent with the Pharmaceutical Care Cycle. The screening has less to do with assessing a patient's needs than with measuring some sort of physiological parameter and suggesting further follow-up by the physician.

Screening programs may also cause confusion with physicians. At first glance, screening programs can appear to be diagnostic in nature. For example, if a screening result suggests that a patient has elevated cholesterol, it can be tempting to interpret this as "needs additional drug therapy" and contact the patient's physician to request a prescription. Pharmacists are strongly cautioned to avoid screening patients in this fashion. Other than for self-limited conditions treated over the counter, pharmacists are not qualified to make a medical diagnosis. The problem of "needs additional drug therapy" is only a valid one after a physician has made a medical diagnosis.

When pharmacists set up new screening programs, they must ensure that patients, physicians, and other stakeholders understand that the programs are intended to identify patients at risk for a health problem so that they can be referred to a qualified physician to receive a diagnosis. It is vital that pharmacists are not the first health care professional to inform a patient they have a particular medical condition. We are qualified to tell a patient his blood pressure is elevated, but not to call that hypertension.

When pharmacists set up new screening programs, they must ensure that patients, physicians, and other stakeholders understand that the programs are intended to identify patients at risk for a health problem so that they can be referred to a qualified physician to receive a diagnosis.

Medication Therapy Management Services (MTMS)

Although the specific services to be offered under MTMS remain under development at this time, one likely scenario is that they will include "brown bag" sessions in which patients bring all their medications to the pharmacist to be reviewed. If the review includes a formal assessment of the patient's needs for drug therapy (appropriate indication, safety, efficacy, compliance, and no untreated indications) then MTMS would be consistent with the practice of pharmaceutical care and the taxonomy of drug therapy problems.

Self Assessment Questions

2.1 In the following patient case, what screening questions should the pharmacist ask to assess if the drug therapy problem has been resolved?

Patient Mildred Janssen takes a combination of warfarin 1 mg and 3 mg tablets for atrial fibrillation. Her dose often changes according to her International Normalized Ratio (INR) and she is confused about how much medication of each strength to take and how often. The pharmacist identified the drug therapy problem as "Inappropriate Compliance."

2.2 Below are four examples of problems that patients may have with their skin. Which are drug therapy problems and which are medical problems? Why?

a. A rash after being exposed to poison ivy.

b. A rash after beginning therapy with lamotrigine.

c. "Red Man Syndrome" after a vancomycin infusion.

d. Psoriasis.

2.3 Rephrase each of the drug therapy problems below to reflect the problem a patient has so that physicians and others will not be confused or offended by the use of pharmacy terminology.

a. Wrong drug: A patient with migraine headaches has been prescribed acetaminophen with codeine 30 mg but is still bothered by painful headaches.

b. Dose too high: A 78-year-old patient presents a new prescription for digoxin 0.25 mg po qd # 30 and her resting pulse rate is 66.

c. Noncompliance: A patient cannot afford to fill a prescription for infliximab for severe Crohn's Disease.

d. Needs additional drug therapy: A patient with chronic persistent asthma is treated only with an albuterol inhaler used as needed.

2.4 Give three examples of drug therapy problems that could be uncovered using traditional profile review and computer screening software. Do pharmacists find drug therapy problems purposefully or accidentally when using these tools?

2.5 Give three examples of drug therapy problems that could *not* be uncovered using traditional profile review and computer screening software. How does interviewing patients help pharmacists search for drug therapy problems?

2.6 For the following cases, what need has not been met and what is the related drug therapy problem?

- Gerald takes 80 mg of simvastatin per day for hyper-lipidemia and his total cholesterol remains elevated. A pill count suggests he takes his medication as instructed but his simvastatin is ineffective.

- Linda (47 years old) has been started on zolpidem 5 mg at bedtime as needed. She wakes up the next morning too groggy to drive to work safely.

- Ted has undiagnosed major depressive disorder. He would meet appropriate criteria for needing drug therapy if he saw a doctor.

- Louis has no prescription insurance and cannot afford the cost of his levodopa/carbidopa and entacapone for Parkinson's Disease, so he takes his medication sporadically to make it last longer.

2.7 For each of the following examples, which patient need is not being met, what is the most likely drug therapy problem, and what is the cause of the drug therapy problem?

a. A woman who is 6 weeks pregnant presents a new prescription for atorvastatin 20 mg daily written by a cardiologist whom she just saw for the first time.

b. A hospitalized patient with moderate renal and hepatic impairment is to begin total parenteral nutrition (TPN). The pharmacist calculates the patient's protein needs at 60 g per day. The prescription order for day 1 of TPN instructs the pharmacy IV room to compound 60 g of amino acids per 24-hour bag.

c. A patient with Parkinson's Disease has tremors that make it nearly impossible to administer his glaucoma eye drops.

d. A child with chronic, persistent asthma is being treated with nebulized albuterol treatments four times daily.

e. An obese patient with blood pressure controlled by felodipine starts the "grapefruit juice" diet.

f. A patient who travels for work keeps his insulin in the car's glove compartment.

g. A patient with migraine headaches presents new prescriptions for zolmitriptan tablets from her family physician and sumatriptan nasal spray from her neurologist.

2.8 Are the following drug therapy problems actual or potential? Why?

a. A patient with a cardiac dysrhythmia who has been stable on amiodarone presents a new prescription for quinidine sulfate.

b. A patient requests a new albuterol inhaler every two or three weeks. The pharmacist determines his inhalation technique is adequate but the patient complains of frequent shortness of breath.

c. A pharmacist offers an osteoporosis screening program. One patient he screens has a t-score of –2.9, suggesting she may have osteoporosis and require additional drug therapy.

2.9 How would these pharmacists communicate potential drug therapy problems if they hope to convince the physician to change drug therapy? If the physician refuses to change the therapy, how would they discuss these potential drug therapy problems with their patients?

a. Fran receives a prescription from Dr. Lattimer for rosuvastatin, the only statin she ever prescribes. Fran knows it's not the safest statin nor is it the drug of choice for most patients.

b. Letricia receives a new prescription from Dr. Garcia for co-trimoxazole for a patient who takes phenytoin for epilepsy. Letricia knows there is potential risk to increase phenytoin toxicity.

2.10 Raquel Uribe has just implemented a cholesterol screening program in her pharmacy. She discusses the results with a patient and since his lipid profile is abnormal, recommends he consult with his primary care provider for follow-up and diagnosis. How should Raquel respond when she receives an angry phone call from Dr. Lipchuk accusing her of practicing medicine without a license?

Reflection Question

Think about a pharmacy practice you have seen or have worked in. How often are drug therapy problems identified in that practice? How did pharmacists identify the drug therapy problems?

References

1. Tomechko MA, Strand LM, Morley PC. Q and A from the pharmaceutical care project in Minnesota. *Am Pharm*.1995;NS35(4):30-9.

2. Currie JD, Chrischilles EA, Kuehl AK, et al. Effect of a training program on community pharmacists' detection of and intervention in drug-related problems. *J Am Pharm Assoc*. 1997;NS37:182-91.

3. Cipolle RJ, Strand LM, Morley PC. *Pharmaceutical Care Practice: The Clinician's Guide*. 2nd ed. New York: McGraw Hill;2004:24-66.

4. Hagel HP, Rovers JP. Consumer education as a cognitive service business development model for pharmacists. August 2, 2006. Available at: http://www.tcpf.org/grants_awarded.php. Accessed August 2, 2006.

5. *Principles of Practice for Pharmaceutical Care*. Washington DC; American Pharmaceutical Association; 1995.

Notes

Patient Data Collection

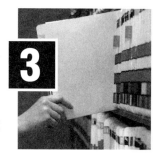

3

John P. Rovers

hapter 2 introduced the concept and taxonomy of drug therapy problems and concluded that the practice of pharmaceutical care is identifying, resolving and preventing such problems. Once pharmacists know what drug therapy problems are, they must go about finding them. To find drug therapy problems, the first thing a pharmacist needs is information about her patient.

This chapter covers history taking and data gathering, including types of data, how data may be collected using patient interviews and other tools, and specific data that are needed to provide pharmaceutical care. First, it will discuss how to sit down with a patient and gather her complete pharmaceutical history. Next the idea of the focused history is presented, when a pharmacist gathers information only on the immediate problem or health issue. Finally, this section discusses how pharmacists can gather patient histories during routine interactions such as patient counseling, drug information questions, or nonprescription medicine recommendations.

Many pharmacists struggle to fit enhanced patient care into an already busy practice. They may also have trouble convincing their owner or manager to implement new patient care programs. For these pharmacists, trying focused or routine care interviews can be a good way to start. These tools are faster and cheaper to implement and can be effective for convincing upper management to enhance the pharmacy's patient care focus. They are a means to get enough information to enter the Pharmaceutical Care Cycle (see Figure 2-1).

Relatively few community pharmacists sit down with a patient for a half-hour, ask him a lot of questions, take copious notes, and fill in lots of forms. Processes like these happen most often in a disease management program in which having a complete picture of a patient's medical and pharmaceutical history is

In this chapter, the following concepts are reviewed:

- Defining subjective and objective information.

- Developing a therapeutic relationship with a patient.

- Deciding which patients must be interviewed.

- Completing an in-depth patient interview.

- Using data collection forms.

necessary to provide quality care. Pharmacists working in ambulatory care clinics or inpatient settings may also gather very thorough patient histories. The new Medicare Part D Medication Therapy Management Services (MTMS) may utilize patient histories to fully assess their drug therapy. As pharmacy faces new reimbursable patient care opportunities, the ability to collect information from patients will become more critical.

The next chapters will discuss how patient data are evaluated in order to identify drug therapy problems and develop care plans. Data collection and evaluation are not separate processes; a pharmacist can gather and assess information at the same time. Eventually she will be able to mentally develop her care plan while gathering and assessing the patient history. For teaching purposes the steps are divided into separate events, but the entire process is a smooth and seamless one. There is a growth curve to learning these patient care skills. However, an experienced practitioner working on a focused problem will complete them very quickly.

Data collection is the first step towards creating a permanent record that can be used for ongoing care of the patient.

Data collection is the first step towards creating a permanent record that can be used for ongoing care of the patient. The initial interview establishes the professional relationship and initiates the patient's pharmacy record. It also helps a pharmacist build a comprehensive database and develop a good working knowledge of the patient's total health picture. Conducting a series of interviews, instead of just one long one, is common in disease management programs. Subsequent interviews should focus on updating existing information and gathering new data.

To collect an accurate, comprehensive patient history there must be a strong professional relationship between pharmacist and patient, characterized by caring, trust, open communication, cooperation, and mutual decision-making. The insightful pharmacist who focuses on the patient, asks good, open-ended questions, and listens attentively will be successful at developing these relationships.

Subjective vs. Objective

Both subjective and objective data are collected as a basis for pharmaceutical care.

Subjective data, such as the patient's medical history, chief complaint, history of the present illness, general health and activity status, and social history are often supplied by the patient. This information cannot be measured directly and may not al-

A PRACTICAL GUIDE TO PHARMACEUTICAL CARE: A Clinical Skills Primer

ways be accurate or reproducible; pharmacists are limited in their ability to confirm the accuracy of data the patient provides.

Objective data can be measured, are observable, and are not influenced by emotion or prejudice. Much objective information is numerical. Examples are vital signs and laboratory measures of substances such as blood lipids.

Generally, if the patient supplied the information, it is more than likely subjective data. Information drawn from a hospital or nursing home chart or obtained directly from the physician's office is generally considered objective. And data drawn from the pharmacy's dispensing computer is objective, but it may be incomplete.

Is a patient's medication history subjective or objective? Many pharmacists consider it to be subjective data since it is usually gathered directly from the patient. Others feel that this information is objective, because it is measurable and pharmacists are the only health care practitioners trained to gather this history. Many practitioners assume compliance data are objective because they assess such information every day. Students are advised to check with their faculty or preceptors to determine any local requirements to consider medication or compliance histories subjective or objective.

Although laboratory data are typically considered to be objective, this depends on the source of the information. If a patient tells the pharmacist that his doctor said his cholesterol is 255 mg/dL, it is not confirmed data so it is subjective. But if the same patient shows a lab results slip, the information is objective. Increasingly pharmacists are collecting their own objective data. Tests for peak expiratory flow rates, blood pressures, serum glucose levels, and serum lipid profiles are now commonly done in the pharmacy to provide the practitioner with truly objective data.

BOX 3-1

Subjective and Objective Data

Pharmaceutical care practitioners collect two types of data to help them evaluate and manage patients' drug therapy: subjective and objective.

Subjective data cannot be measured directly and may not always be accurate or reproducible. Most of the data that the pharmacist collects directly from patients, such as medical history, are subjective.

Objective data are measurable and observable, and are not influenced by emotion or prejudice. Much objective information is numerical.

Sometimes pharmacists are surprised to find that they do not have any objective data recorded after taking a patient history. Not all patient care requires objective data. It is important to record that the pharmacist attempted to gather this information, but none was relevant to the patient's care.

A final type of data can be characterized as "objective, but incomplete." An example is data collected simply by looking at a computerized dispensing record. Although the computer record is certainly objective and accurate with respect to prescription products filled and refilled at that pharmacy, most of the time it will not include nonprescription medications, physician samples, medications received elsewhere, etc. It is not fully useful until the pharmacist gathers a more thorough history.

Pharmacists need not be overly concerned whether medication histories, compliance data, or laboratory values are subjective or objective. What type of data to collect is more important than how it is organized. For the sake of simplicity, many practitioners consider medication histories and compliance data to be subjective, and lab tests to be objective, regardless of the source. Students are advised to consult with their faculty and preceptors to determine how they would like to see such information handled.

The Therapeutic Relationship

The therapeutic relationship is a shared responsibility between the patient and the pharmacist, who agree to work together to bring about the best results possible. The therapeutic relationship is usually entered into at the stage in the Pharmaceutical Care Cycle where the pharmacist qualifies the patient to receive care (see Figure 2-1).

A therapeutic relationship is one in which the patient will freely share with the pharmacist information that he might find embarrassing or potentially damaging. Pharmacists are obliged to use such information only in the direct care of a patient and must keep it completely confidential.

Without a therapeutic relationship, none of the steps necessary to provide pharmaceutical care can occur. Many patients are already uncomfortable with sharing personal health information with their insurers. If they do not understand why a pharmacist is collecting information or do not believe that the information will be used only to help them, they will at best edit the information they provide the pharmacist and, at worst, refuse the pharmacist's offer of care altogether. They may even lie if they find the questions too intrusive.

Most of the information needed to provide pharmaceutical care must be gathered from the patient. But sometimes patients might not want to share information that the pharmacist needs to help them. This may be because many pharmacists and patients have had a cordial business relationship more often than a health care relationship. And the wide variety of general merchandise for sale in many community pharmacies suggests a retail environment, not a health care setting. When patients view pharmacists as retailers instead of health care professionals, they may be unwilling to share their sensitive health information.

The therapeutic relationship is a shared responsibility between the patient and the pharmacist, who agree to work together to bring about the best results possible.

Pharmacists working in health systems, ambulatory care clinics, or practicing long-term care may find it easier to enter into a therapeutic relationship. Patients who receive care in such settings only see the pharmacist in the role of health care professional. This can make patients more likely to place their trust in the pharmacist. For pharmacists who do work in a traditional community setting, installing a private or semiprivate consultation area may send a subtle message that the pharmacy is a patient care setting as well as a place of business. Patients will appreciate being able to discuss their personal information where other patrons cannot hear.

In a therapeutic relationship, patients recognize that the pharmacist is a health care provider. A good way to initiate the therapeutic relationship is for her to say something like this: "At this pharmacy we do things a little differently. For me to help you the best I can, I need to ask you some questions that you may not have been asked before by a pharmacist. I appreciate that some

---

BOX 3-2

Confidential versus Private

Keeping information private means telling no one about it. Keeping it confidential means only sharing it with other providers who need that information to care for the patient. There will be times when it will be necessary to share patient information with the patient's physician, nurse, or another pharmacist.

Patients and others sometimes misunderstand the Health Insurance Portability and Accountability Act (HIPAA). Pharmacists and others are permitted to share a patient's health information in order to provide patient care. It may be wise to inform patients of how you will use their health information at the time you gather their histories.

Which Patients Should Be Interviewed?

When pharmacists want to move into pharmaceutical care and start interviewing their patients, they are immediately faced with a dilemma: Whom should they interview? Often, there is no good way to tell. Without interviewing patients and gathering more data, they will only do a partial job of patient care because many drug therapy problems are not immediately apparent.

In the community setting, most drug therapy problems are seen with refill prescriptions, so concentrating on those patients and keeping interviews narrowly focused may save time.

In the health system or nursing home setting, targeting efforts to certain high-risk groups of patients (e.g., those receiving anticoagulation therapy or with a history of falls) may be an efficient means to qualify patients to receive pharmaceutical care.

---

of this may be rather new, but please rest assured that this information is completely confidential and will only be used to help us both make decisions about your health care."

The pharmacist may not need a patient's explicit permission to gather data, but should make sure she has his cooperation. She must be attentive to body language or facial expressions that suggest the patient is uncomfortable with the interview process. Demonstrating caring will be the most valuable tool towards developing this relationship.

The Patient Interview

The patient interview is critical because it provides the pharmacist with necessary information used to identify drug therapy problems, make drug therapy decisions, and develop a care plan. Through the interview, the following subjective and objective data are collected:

• Demographic information, including patients' financial and insurance status.

• General health and activity status, including diet, exercise, and social information.

• Chief complaint.

• History of present illness.

• Past medical history.

- Medication history including all prescription drugs, samples, nonprescription medications, herbals, and nutritional products.

- Patients' thoughts or feelings and perceptions of their condition or disease, including their desired outcome and preferred means used to achieve that outcome.

The information must be timely, accurate, and complete; organized and recorded to assure that it is readily retrievable; updated as necessary; and maintained in a confidential manner. Most information can be gathered by talking with and observing the patient, but the interview should be organized and professional. The interview must be confidential and private, and should be long enough to ensure that questions and answers can be fully developed.

The ability to gather a complete history is a critical skill, especially when a patient is seeking pharmaceutical care services but does not have a particular complaint. Pharmacists in office-based practices or who market their services as medication check-ups may find themselves in this situation. Without any guidance on where to start helping the patient, a thorough history is mandatory. A complete history is also useful when providing Medicare Part D MTMS.

Effective Interpersonal Interactions in Interviews

Successful interpersonal interactions with patients rely on two basic skills: good communication and accurate information gathering. The first step in beginning a patient interview is for the pharmacist to introduce himself, smile, and shake hands firmly. He should explain the interviewing process to the patient honestly and directly. Communicating warmth and welcome to the patient is important, as is establishing friendly eye contact.

The pharmacist can direct the patient to the consultation area if there is one, or move to a less crowded area where interruptions are unlikely. Using statements like "Please have a seat over here," instead of, "Would you like to have a seat?" helps pharmacists be assertive in a nonthreatening way. Although not an explicit request for permission to proceed, this does allow the patient to decline the offer of a chair. The pharmacist should interpret this action as hesitation at proceeding further, and should proceed slowly and cautiously while being attentive to the patient's concerns.

Next the pharmacist should explain in more detail exactly what will happen during the patient interview. A brief overview of the pharmaceutical care process may be necessary to put the interview in context. In the interest of establishing a trusting relationship, the pharmacist may want to explain why patient information is needed, how it will be stored, and how it will be used in patient care.

The pharmacist should indicate how long the interview will last and respect the patient's schedule; it's important to ensure that it is a convenient time to conduct the interview. If it isn't, he should schedule an appointment later.

A friendly, professional tone is a must. The pharmacist's words and manner should convey that he is a health care professional collecting necessary data.

Body language of both patient and pharmacist is important, because much communication is nonverbal. Body language that indicates warmth and interest includes friendly eye contact (not staring), leaning towards the other person, and maintaining a pleasant, concerned facial expression. Signals of discomfort, fear, or anger include avoiding eye contact, turning the body away from the other person, crossing arms, or maintaining a neutral or negative facial expression.

To get the most complete answers possible, pharmacists should ask open-ended questions that begin with the words "who," "what," "where," "when," "why," and "how." Open-ended questions encourage higher-level, synthesized thinking and a wide range of responses. Closed-ended questions, which simply require a "yes" or "no" answer, encourage rote recall of data and a very narrow range of answers.

For example, instead of asking a closed-ended question, such as, "Is this the only medication you are taking?" a pharmacist could ask an open-ended question, such as, "What medications are you currently taking?" This way the pharmacist encourages the patient to reflect on the question, and is more likely to get an accurate answer.

BOX 3-4

Timing, Convenience, and Appointments with Patients

The best time to conduct a patient interview is as soon as a problem is suspected or at the time when the patient requests the pharmacist's assistance. If this is not convenient for either the patient or the pharmacist, they can schedule an interview later, to take place in the pharmacy, over the telephone, via e-mail or even in the patient's home. Another option is to perform a rapid screening interview immediately and then follow up later.

The pharmacist should also make sure that patients are given enough time to respond and think through the question. Common communication mistakes include compound questions, where the questioner links two or more questions together. For example, "What happened after you started taking furosemide? Did you have to get up during the night to urinate?" It is important to wait for the patient to answer the first question before asking the second one.

Another mistake is the leading question in which the listener can tell that the questioner believes there is a right and a wrong answer to the question,   For example, "You did not take more pain pills than prescribed, did you?" Not only is this a closed-ended question, the phrasing makes it clear the correct answer is "No." To avoid a leading question, pharmacists should try not to let biases become evident and maintain a neutral tone in their voices and wording.

The interview can begin with broad questions, and then get more specific. This allows the patient to follow a train of thought.

TABLE 3-1

Tips for Good Interviews: A Summary

To ensure an interview is effective and runs smoothly, pharmacists should:

* Greet the patient.

* Explain the interviewing process.

* Direct the patient to the consultation area if you have one.

* Introduce the interview process in more detail.

* Indicate how long the interview will last.

* Use words and manners that convey professionalism.

* Pay attention to body language.

* Ask open-ended questions.

* Give patients adequate time for responses.

* Use good listening skills.

* Use a list of questions as a prompt.

* Ask the patient to restate any unclear information.

* Communicate at the appropriate educational level and avoid medical jargon.

Sometimes, it may be necessary to prompt patients to supply more specific information about a symptom or problem.

When some pharmacists interview patients they rely on a list of questions called the "Basic Seven" (see Table 3-2). They may even keep the list handy on a laminated card.[1] Responses to the Basic Seven will usually guide the pharmacist either to identify the drug therapy problem and a possible solution or refer the patient to a physician for medical evaluation.

In addition to using the Basic Seven for screening, three questions developed by the U.S. Public Health Service are useful to determine how well patients understand their drug therapy.[2] They are:

• What did your physician tell you this medication was for?

• How did your physician tell you to use this medication?

• What did your physician tell you to expect from this medication?

These 10 questions provide the pharmacist with considerable patient-specific information. The Basic Seven screening questions give clues about a patient's need for medication, how well the medications are working, possible adverse effects and drug interactions and their severity, possible causative factors for symptoms, and what the patient has already done to alleviate symptoms. These questions also provide the type of data that the physician will need to decide how to act on a pharmacist's

TABLE 3-2

The "Basic Seven" Questions

The Basic Seven screening questions for interviewing include the following:

• **Location:** "Where is the symptom/problem?"

• **Quality:** "What is it like?"

• **Quantity:** "How severe is it?"

• **Timing:** "How long or how often has it been present?"

• **Setting:** "How did it happen?"

• **Modifying Factors:** "What makes it better? Worse?"

• **Associated Symptoms:** "What other symptoms do you have?"

recommendation. The three Public Health Service questions are especially useful during medication counseling sessions because they may provide evidence that a patient has a potential problem with compliance. If the pharmacist calls the doctor without answers to the Basic Seven, the physician will usually ask to see the patient.

Although these 10 questions generate valuable information, they are screening questions only and are not an adequate substitute for a well-taken history. If patients do not complain of symptoms, the Basic Seven screening questions may be insufficient to indicate whether the patient has a drug therapy problem. Note that all 10 questions are open-ended; additional follow-up questions should be more narrowly focused. Eventually, closed-ended questions may be used to definitively identify the drug therapy problems.

Concentrating on the patient's descriptions should be the pharmacist's focus. To listen as effectively as possible, she should minimize environmental distractions such as noise and nearby store traffic. Common barriers to listening include:

• Thinking about what one will say next.

• Trying to do two things at once.

• Jumping to conclusions.

• Interrupting the speaker.

Using a list of questions to guide the interview prevents having to think about what to say while the patient is speaking. It may be necessary to tape record the interview so as not to get caught in the "note-taking rather than listening" trap. Pharmacists can practice focusing on the patient's actual words instead of forecasting the patient's response and interrupting.

To ensure that the information recorded is correct, the pharmacist should ask the patient to restate any unclear information. The pharmacist should briefly restate the patient's words if she is not sure what is meant.

Communicating at the appropriate educational level is important. Pharmacists should avoid medical terminology or jargon unless they are positive that the patient understands it. Talking over a patient's head does not encourage an open patient care relationship.

Other Information to Collect

Pharmacists may want to compile other material to supplement information gathered from the patient interview, such as other pharmacy records, the patient's medical record or medical reports, comments from the patient's family, and input from the patient's other health care providers, including physicians and other pharmacies. The pharmacist may also need to use physical assessment techniques, such as blood pressure monitoring or blood glucose testing, to acquire patient-specific objective information.

Using Data Collection Forms

An old axiom says that patients will say what is wrong with them if they are asked the right questions. With training and persistence, pharmacists can learn to ask the right questions. With practice, they not only become faster, but interviews become much more useful and the data collected more consistent.

Beginners just developing their interview skills often inquire first about the patient's medication history, and may move on to a question about a lab test in the physician's office, a query into the patient's social history, or another question about medication. This approach can confuse patients, who often have no idea what the pharmacist wants to know. As a result, some patients will answer questions as narrowly as possible and others provide all manner of information, relevant and otherwise. Neither is helpful to the pharmacist.

For pharmacists to get patients to share information in a useful way, they need to make the sharing easy. Many have found data collection forms to be helpful tools. A data collection form gathers related questions together so they may be asked at the same time. A well-designed form will include space for a pharmacist to record information related to:

• Basic patient demographics.

• Prescription and nonprescription drug use.

• Social and family history.

• Medical history.

• Complaints or symptoms that indicate how well drug therapy is working.

- Possible adverse effects or potential untreated conditions that require the pharmacist's intervention or referral to a physician.

Patients can complete the form while waiting for their prescriptions to be filled. In a health system or ambulatory clinic setting, the patient can complete the form in the waiting area before their appointment. Pharmacists should explain the nature of the form and why the information is being requested. Later, during interviews, they can review the form with patients and clarify and expand on sections that suggest a problem exists. Sometimes, for example, a patient may simply circle an entire column of "no" answers with a single pen stroke—thus the pharmacist should investigate further.

Pharmacists should make sure patients read each question, understand it, and provide a complete, accurate answer. Then they should avoid asking all those same questions again when reviewing the form. If they do, patients are likely to wonder why the pharmacist had them complete the form in the first place. Time with the patient is used to fill in gaps and expand upon the form.

Alternatively pharmacists can complete the form during a formal patient interview, possibly gathering more and better information because they can ask follow-up questions. This may also be a better approach for developing the therapeutic relationship.

Commonly used data collection forms are shown in Figures 3-1, 3-2, 3-3, 3-4 and 3-5. These forms are useful for data collection and history taking, and they also help establish a chart for each patient. A patient chart is necessary for pharmacists to keep each patient's information properly organized.

Figures 3-4 and 3-5 were originally developed by clinical faculty working in an inpatient and long-term care setting, respectively. In addition to being useful data collection tools, these forms also act as patient monitoring forms.

The Patient History Form in Figure 3-1 lends itself to being completed by the patient and reviewed with the pharmacist. It is quite short, looks similar to other forms the patient is used to filling in, and inquires into all facets of the patient's history necessary to provide pharmaceutical care.

The Patient History Form also includes a place for the pharmacist or the patient to indicate the effectiveness of a drug. This is very useful data to determine if a patient has had a positive or negative outcome and to identify possible drug therapy problems. Either the pharmacist or the patient can complete the one-page Pharmaceutical Care History Form (Figure 3-2). The supplementary Medication History and Medical History Form (Figure 3-3) is best completed by the pharmacist during the patient interview. This form is longer than the others and includes suggested questions regarding previous adverse effects, compliance, and the patient's ability to afford medications.

On the forms in Figure 3-1 and Figure 3-2, there is a place for the patient to circle a large number of clinical complaints and other conditions. Pharmacist should pay special attention to anything the patient has circled with a "yes," and ask herself if a drug caused the problem or if a drug will be needed to fix it. Often, this answer indicates a drug therapy problem. Sometimes it means the patient requires additional drug therapy, and sometimes it indicates an adverse effect or drug interaction.

The form in Figure 3-4 was developed by a clinical pharmacist working in a health system and is appropriate for use in most inpatient care settings. The front of the page provides space for a medication history and the necessary monitoring parameters. At the bottom of the front page are several reminders for the pharmacist to ensure appropriate prophylactic measures for the critically ill. The back of the page provides space to monitor the patient's progress.

The form in Figure 3-5 was developed for use in the long-term care setting. The front page provides space to link medications to specific diagnoses and reminds the pharmacist to adjust the dose for renal impairment if required. The back of the page allows for various laboratory results plus ongoing clinical and therapeutic drug monitoring, especially for glucose and warfarin which must often be monitored intensely.

Unlike Figures 3-1, 3-2 and 3-3, Figures 3-4 and 3-5 are specifically designed for ongoing patient monitoring and patient history data collection. These can be useful when following patients over time. As new information is gathered in follow-up sessions, it can be added quickly and efficiently.

The form in Figure 3-6, the Pharmaceutical Care Data Sheet, is an abbreviated form that has been found to be useful if only a brief or informal encounter is possible, or if the patient wants to treat a condition with a nonprescription medication. (Patients requiring a nonprescription medication have a drug therapy problem by definition and may be ideal candidates for pharmaceutical

FIGURE 3-1

Patient History Form

PATIENT HISTORY FORM

Name: _____ Date: _____

Mailing Address: _____

| Street | city | state | zip |

Social Security Number: _____ Phone: (H) _____ (W) _____

DOB: _____ Height: _____ Weight: _____ HR: _____ BP: _____

Gender: _____ Pregnancy Status: _____

Allergies: _____ **Reactions:** _____

PRESCRIPTION MEDICATION HISTORY						
Name/Strength	Directions	Start Date	Stop Date	Physician	Purpose	Effectiveness

NONPRESCRIPTION USE: Check conditions for which you have used a nonprescription medication.

____headache	____drowsiness	____heartburn/GI upset/gas
____eye/ear problems	____weight loss	____vitamins
____cold/flu	____diarrhea	____herbal products
____allergies	____hemorrhoids	____organic products
____sinus	____muscle/joint pain	____other: _____
____cough	____rash/itching/dry skin	
____sleeplessness		

NONPRESCRIPTION MEDICATION HISTORY					
Name/Strength	Directions	Purpose	How Often	Effectiveness	

FIGURE 3-1

Patient History Form, continued

MEDICAL PROBLEMS: Have you experienced, or do you have: (circle Y or N)

known kidney problems?	Y N	sores on legs or feet?	Y N
frequent urinary infections?	Y N	known blood clot problems?	Y N
difficulty with urination?	Y N	leg pain or swelling?	Y N
frequent urination at night?	Y N	unusual bleeding or bruising?	Y N
known liver problems/hepatitis?	Y N	anemia?	Y N
trouble eating certain foods?	Y N	thyroid problems?	Y N
nausea or vomiting?	Y N	known hormone problems?	Y N
constipation or diarrhea?	Y N	arthritis or joint problems?	Y N
bloody or black bowel movements?	Y N	muscle cramps or weakness?	Y N
abdominal pain or cramps?	Y N	memory problems?	Y N
frequent heartburn/indigestion?	Y N	dizziness?	Y N
stomach ulcers in the past?	Y N	hearing or visual problems?	Y N
shortness of breath?	Y N	frequent headaches?	Y N
coughing up phlegm or blood?	Y N	rash or hives?	Y N
chest pain or tightness?	Y N	change in appetite/taste?	Y N
fainting spells or passing out?	Y N	walking/balance problems?	Y N
thumping or racing heart?	Y N	other problems?	Y N

MEDICAL HISTORY: Have you or any blood relative had: (mark all that apply)

	self	relative		self	relative
high blood pressure	__	__	heart disease	__	__
asthma	__	__	stroke	__	__
cancer	__	__	kidney disease	__	__
depression	__	__	mental illness	__	__
lung disease	__	__	substance abuse	__	__
diabetes	__	__	other _____		

SOCIAL HISTORY: Please indicate your tobacco, alcohol, caffeine, and dietary habits

Nicotine Use
____ never smoked
____ packs per day for ____ Years
____ stopped ____ year(s) ago

Caffeine Intake
____ never consumed
____ drinks per day
____ stopped ____ years(s) ago

Alcohol Consumption
____ never consumed
____ drinks per day/week
____ stopped ____ year(s) ago

Diet Restrictions/Patterns
____ number of meals per day
____ food restrictions:_____
_____

OTHER INFORMATION/COMMENTS:

FIGURE 3-2

Pharmaceutical Care History Form

Pharmaceutical Care History

Name:_____ Date:_____

Allergies: (include medicines and foods):_____
_____

Unwanted Medicine Effects in the Past: _____
_____

Smoking History: _____never smoked   _____stopped smoking
                 _____packs per day for_____years

Alcohol History: _____never drank   _____stopped drinking
                 _____drinks per day for_____years

Other drug use: (caffeine, marijuana, etc.) _____
_____

How many meals do you eat each day?_____

What special food or diet restriction do you have?_____

Height:_____Weight:_____

Family History:

Have you or any blood relative had: (mark all that apply)

	self	relative		self	relative
alcoholism	___	___	stroke	___	___
asthma	___	___	high blood pressure	___	___
cancer	___	___	kidney disease	___	___
depression	___	___	mental illness	___	___
diabetes	___	___	other conditions_____		
heart disease	___	___	_____		
lung disease	___	___	_____		

Present Medical Problems:

Have you experienced, or do you have: (circle Y or N)

known kidney problems?	Y N	sores on legs or feet?	Y N
frequent urinary infections?	Y N	known blood clot problems?	Y N
difficulty with urination?	Y N	leg pain or swelling?	Y N
frequent urination at night?	Y N	unusual bleeding or bruising?	Y N
known liver problems/hepatitis?	Y N	anemia?	Y N
trouble eating certain foods?	Y N	thyroid problems?	Y N
nausea or vomiting?	Y N	known hormone problems?	Y N
constipation or diarrhea?	Y N	arthritis or joint pain?	Y N
bloody or black bowel movements?	Y N	muscle cramps or weakness?	Y N
abdominal pain or cramps?	Y N	memory problems?	Y N
frequent heartburn/indigestion?	Y N	dizziness?	Y N
stomach ulcers in the past?	Y N	hearing or visual problems?	Y N
shortness of breath?	Y N	frequent headaches?	Y N
coughing up of phlegm or blood?	Y N	rash or hives?	Y N
chest pain or tightness?	Y N	change in appetite/taste?	Y N
fainting spells or passing out?	Y N	walking or balance problems?	Y N
thumping or racing heart?	Y N	other problems?_____	

All information is confidential. Thank you for completing this form. We will use it to better care for you.

63

FIGURE 3-3

Medication History and Medical History Form

Medication History and Medical History Form

| Ht   Wt | | Sex   Birth Date | | LBW | | Race |
Name

I. Data Collection Collected By:

Interview Start: Stop:

Date:

Prescribed Medications

Name/Strength	Dose	Duration	Purpose	Efficacy	ADRs	Dr.	Comment

Prescribed Medications Not Currently Taking or Historical Medications

Dose/Strength	Dose	Duration	Purpose	Dr.	Why Not Still Taking

FIGURE 3-3

Medication History and Medical History Form, continued

Nonprescription Medications

Name/Strength	Dose	Duration	Purpose	Efficacy	ADRs	Dr.	Comment::

Completion of nonprescription medication history
    What do you take for the following conditions?
    (enter on OTC list, ask follow-up questions)
        headache
        cold/flu
        allergies
        sinus
        cough
        sleeplessness
        drowsiness
        weight loss
        heartburn/stomach upset/gas
        constipation
        diarrhea
        hemorrhoids
        muscle or joint pain
        rash/itching/dry skin/skin problems

        vitamins/minerals
        herbal products/home remedies/health food store products
        natural/organic products
        other
        caffeine
        alcohol
        tobacco
        illicit drugs

FIGURE 3-3

Medication History and Medical History Form, continued

History Collection Form, Page - 3 Patient Name. _____

What medication allergies do you have? (drug name, type of reaction)

What environmental allergies do you have?

What type of adverse (bad) reactions have you had to medications in the past?

Compliance assessment
Base questions on history obtained to this point.
Your medication regimen sounds complex and must be hard to follow; how often would you estimate that you miss a dose?
Everyone has problems with following a medication regimen exactly as written. What are the problems you are having with your regimen?

Payment/Reimbursement Issues
How much of a problem are medication/treatment costs?

Completion of Medical History

    What other diagnoses (conditions) do you have that we haven't already covered?

Diagnosis	Onset Date	Comments	

Which problems are currently active, or still a problem for you?

Pertinent ROS

FIGURE 3-4

Critical Care Pharmacotherapy Monitoring Sheet

Patient Pharmacotherapy Monitoring

Patient Name:	Age:	Ht:
Medical Record No:	Sex:	Wt:
Allergies:	Room:	IBW:
	Admit Date:	CrCl:

Scheduled Medications	PRN Medications	Medical Problem List
1.	1.	
2.	2.	
3.	3.	
4.	4.	
5.	5.	
6.	6.	
7.	7.	
8.	8.	
9.	9.	
10.	10.	
11.	11.	
12.	12.	
13.	13.	
14.	14.	

Home Medications	PMH	Labs
1.		Date: T P R BP
2.		
3.		
4.		
5.		
6.		
7.		
8.		
9.		
10.		
11.		
12.		
13.		
14.	EtOH	
15.	Tobacco	

HPI	Culture Results			Notes
	Date	Site	Results	

Steroid Coverage
DVT Prophylaxis
Stress Ulcer Prophylaxis
Antibiotics

Nutrition
Tube Feed & Rate
TPN & Rate
MD

FIGURE 3-4

Critical Care Pharmacotherapy Monitoring Sheet, continued

| Date: | T | P | R | BP | | Date: | T | P | R | BP |

Other Labs/PE:

Other Labs/PE:

Medication Changes			Medication Changes	
1.	5.		1.	5.
2.	6.		2.	6.
3.	7.		3.	7.
4.	8.		4.	8.

Notes:

Notes:

| Date: | T | P | R | BP | | Date: | T | P | R | BP |

Other Labs/PE:

Other Labs/PE:

Medication Changes			Medication Changes	
1.	5.		1.	5.
2.	6.		2.	6.
3.	7.		3.	7.
4.	8.		4.	8.

Notes:

Notes:

| Date: | T | P | R | BP | | Date: | T | P | R | BP |

Other Labs/PE:

Other Labs/PE:

Medication Changes			Medication Changes	
1.	5.		1.	5.
2.	6.		2.	6.
3.	7.		3.	7.
4.	8.		4.	8.

Notes:

Notes:

FIGURE 3-5

Geriatric Pharmacotherapy Monitoring Form

Geriatric Pharmacotherapy Monitoring Form

Pt Location:		Date of Review:		Prescriber:	
Pt Name:			D.O.B.:	Age:	Gender: M / F
Ht:	ABW:		IBW:		CrCl:
Social History	Tobacco:			EtOH:	
Family History					

Allergies:

Diagnosis List		
1.	7.	13.
2.	8.	14.
3.	9.	15.
4.	10.	16.
5.	11.	17.
6.	12.	18.

Current Medications				
Start	Medication	Diag. #	Renal Adj.	Monitoring

FIGURE 3-5

Geriatric Pharmacotherapy Monitoring Form, continued

Date		Date	

Other Labs/PE: Other Labs/PE:

BP: Pulse   BP: Pulse

Date		Date	

Other Labs/PE: Other Labs/PE:

BP: Pulse   BP: Pulse

Albumin:	B12	Folate:	PSA:	TSH:

Lipids		Iron Studies		Liver Enzymes	
CHO:	HDL:	Fe:	Ferritin:	SGOT/AST	AlkPo4:
TGY:	LDL:	TIBC:	Fe Sat:	SGPT/ALT:	

Glucose Monitoring HbAlc/Date					
Accucheck Date/Time					

Warfarin Monitoring					
Date INR Dose					

Serum Drug Concentrations				
Drug	Date	Time	Level	Normal Range

Courtesy of Kristin S. Meyer, PharmD, CGP Drake University and Robert F. Richardson, MS, PharmD, CGP University of Arkansas for Medical Sciences.

FIGURE 3-6

Pharmaceutical Care Data Sheet

Pharmaceutical Care Data Sheet

Date: _____   R.Ph. _____

Pt Name: _____   Allergies _____

_____

Medications: _____   Diagnoses: _____

Drug Therapy Problems:

Notes:

Follow-up: _____   Recorded: _____

FIGURE 3-7

Authorization to Release Medical Information Form

1

Authorization To Release Medical Information

Date_____   Name:_____

2   Date of Birth:_____

                                     SS No.:_____ **3**

                                     Address:_____

                                     Record Number:_____

I, the undersigned, do hereby grant permission for the above named pharmacy to obtain from, release to:

_____

(Name of Person or Institution)

4

_____

(Address)

the following information from the patient's clinical record:

_____

_____ **5**

_____

I understand that this information will be used for the purpose of:

❑ providing information to allow pharmaceutical care to be provided to the patient.

❑ providing information to the physician regarding the care provided by the pharmacist.

❑ supporting the payment of an insurance claim.

❑ other _____

_____ **6**

This authorization will be valid for the period of twelve months unless otherwise specified below. **7**

Release authorized for _____ days   months (circle one)

I understand that I may revoke this consent at any time by sending a written notice to the above named pharmacy. I understand that any release which has been made prior to my revocation and which was made in reliance upon this authorization shall not constitute a breach of my rights to confidentiality. I understand that I may review the disclosed information by contacting the above named pharmacy.

_____   _____

Signature of Patient or Patient's Authorized Representative   Relationship of Authorized Representative

8

_____   _____

Date   Pharmacy Representative/Date

Specific authorization for release of information protected by state or federal law

I specifically authorize the release of data and information relating to:

❑ Substance Abuse   ❑ Mental Health

❑ AIDS/HIV-related information | **PROHIBITION ON REDISCLOSURE**

9 | This form does not authorize redisclosure of

_____ | medical information beyond the limits of this

Signature of Patient or Patient's Authorized Representative/Date | consent. Where information has been disclosed

| from records protected by federal law for alcohol/

| drug abuse records, by state law for mental health

In order for the above information to be released, | records or HIV/AIDS related records, federal

you must sign here and above. | requirements (42 CFR Part 2) and state

| requirements (Iowa Code chs. 228/141) prohibit

❑ Release mailed or information sent | further disclosure without the specific written

| consent of the patient, or as otherwise permitted

10 | by such law and/or regulations. A general

_____ | authorization for the release of medical or other

Signature of Patient or Patient's Authorized Representative/Date | information is not sufficient for these purposes.

| Civil and/or criminal penalties may attach for

Original - Pharmacy / Copy - Patient | unauthorized disclosure of alcohol/drug abuse,

8/2/95 | mental health, or HIV/AIDS information.

FIGURE 3-7

Authorization to Release Medical Information Form, continued

Authorization To Release Medical Information, continued

Instructions for use of "Authorization to Release Medical Information" Form

This form is intended to be used when you want to either receive information from, or release information to, other care providers. It has been reviewed by the Iowa Pharmacists Association legal counsel.

Following are suggestions for how to most appropriately use this form. Each of the numbers indicates an area of the form on the attached document.

1. Enter your pharmacy name, address, and phone number.

2. Enter the date the form was completed.

3. Enter necessary patient-identifying information. This is mainly so the receiver of the form can send you the information on the correct patient.

4. Enter name and address of the health care professional or health care facility that you will be contacting. Be sure to check the box indicating whether you are gaining permission to send to, or receive from, that health care provider.

5. Enter a description of the information you are asking to receive from, or send to, the patient's health care provider. For example: vital signs, diagnosis, lab results.

6. Check the box that tells the patient or health care provider the purposes of this need for or use of information. For example: provide pharmaceutical care to the patient.

7. Enter the number of months that this release authorization will be valid, if you or the patient require it to be different than 12 months.

8. Enter signature of patient or patient representative; relationship to patient if patient representative is authorizing; date; and signature of pharmacy representative and date.

9. Check appropriate box if the information includes or requests information relating to substance abuse, mental health, or AIDS/HIV. Enter signature date and signature of patient or patient's representative. The patient or patient representative must sign and date here as well as in section 8.

10. Check box, enter signature date and signature when you send request for information, or send information to health care provider.

care.) Some pharmacists bind these forms into small pads that are easily accessible when patients need assistance. If the patient's name and telephone number are also recorded on the form, it gives the pharmacist a convenient tool for follow-up care to assure that the problem has been alleviated. This form is also useful when undertaking a focused or routine care patient interview.

Data collection forms are good tools for learning how to take a patient history. However, they are intrinsically incomplete and restrictive and may interfere with the pharmacist's listening to the patient. So, most pharmacists use forms less once history-taking becomes an ingrained skill.

Patient Information Release Form

Most of the information that pharmacists collect, either with or without a form, is subjective. Although some objective information can be gathered in the pharmacy, such as lipid profiles or vital signs, the source of objective data is typically the patient's physician or, sometimes, a hospital or clinic.

Pharmacists may call physicians' offices to request information about patients. If the relationship between the pharmacist and physician has historically been one of mutual assistance, co-operation, and respect, the office may provide the information. Physicians who do not know the pharmacist or are not educated about the practice of pharmaceutical care may refuse to provide the requested information, saying that it is confidential.

The Health Insurance Portability and Accountability Act of 1996 (HIPAA) has made both health care providers and patients more sensitive to issues of patient privacy.[3] In the current practice environment, pharmacists should expect that some physicians or other providers may be hesitant to release confidential information even if they understand why the pharmacist needs it. In cases where a pharmacist cannot readily obtain information needed to care for a patient, an appropriately signed release form is invaluable to gain access to the necessary information.

A release form is a legal document that gives an institution or provider formal permission to release certain information to another party, such as the pharmacist. A sample of a patient release form is shown in Figure 3-7. (This form has been reviewed by a lawyer and is legal for use in the state of Iowa.) Pharmacists interested in using a release form are urged to contact qualified legal sources in their own states to ensure that the form they intend to use is legally binding.

When using a release form, pharmacists must be sure to request only the information they absolutely require, such as the results of specific laboratory tests. Requests for "all information" will likely be returned to the pharmacist. When contacting a hospital, it is often useful to request only a copy of the admission history and physical and the discharge summary. These are fairly brief documents that succinctly summarize the patient's stay in the hospital. Be aware that hospitals are often especially sensitive to issues of confidentiality.

It is important to send the form to the person or department that created the data desired. For instance, a laboratory test result should be requested from the lab that performed the test. This will help avoid unnecessary conflicts in the release of patient information. If in doubt, the medical records department should be able to provide guidance as to the appropriate contact person or department.

Specific Data to Collect

This section discusses the specific data elements that are included in a comprehensive patient history. It is rarely necessary to ask for every data element listed here. Pharmacists must edit their questions and focus on the areas that are most relevant.

Before gathering data, pharmacists should determine how the information they request will help assist the patient.

Before gathering data, pharmacists should determine how the information they request will help assist the patient. For example, questions related to substance abuse may be useful to a pharmacist caring for a patient taking disulfiram, but are less relevant for a patient who only drinks occasionally.

At minimum, the history should include the patient's basic demographics, abbreviated social history, medication and disease state histories, and a summary of the present illness. A history consisting of all of the patient's medical conditions, all medications taken, and the clinical effects of all medications may suffice as a tool to rapidly screen for drug therapy problems. If time is sufficient a more comprehensive history can be performed.

Demographic Data

The patient's name, address, home and work telephone numbers, the best time to call, birth date, gender, ethnicity, height, and weight are key demographic data to gather. Some people may be sensitive about sharing some of this information, so pharmacists may wish to indicate why it is needed. For example, African Americans and Asian Americans may metabolize medication at a different rate than Caucasians. When patients will not provide their height and weight, for example, pharmacists should indicate an estimate.

General Appearance and Health Status

Useful information in this category includes the patient's overall appearance and affect; diet, exercise, and sleep habits; if she is pregnant (include due date) or breastfeeding; and if he uses any medical aids or devices such as a wheelchair, pacemaker, or contact lenses.

Social History

This information, which includes the patient's occupation; tobacco, alcohol, and caffeine use; and economic and insurance status helps the pharmacist assess how well a patient will be able to comply with a potential care plan. If a pharmacist does not appreciate the circumstances under which a patient lives, she may devise a care plan that the patient is unable to follow.

Social history also provides clues about the patient's living arrangements that are useful in deciding if a care plan is likely to be successful. For example, if a woman works nights and has difficulty sleeping during the day, recommending pseudoephedrine may not be a wise course because the medication may cause insomnia.

In collecting information on caffeine use, remember that soft drinks, tea, and chocolate are also forms of caffeine. On occasion it may be necessary to get information on illicit drug use and sexual history, but such circumstances are rare. Questions related to these topics, and alcohol use as well, may be poorly received by the patient unless pharmacists first indicate why they need the information.

Having a pharmacist request a social history will be new for most patients and they may not view the pharmacist as a health care provider who needs this type of information to do her job. Pharmacists must respect the wishes of patients who choose not to supply this type of data.

Medication History

Medication history forms one of two central portions of the pharmacist's patient database. A thorough medication history must include significantly more than a simple list of drugs. The pharmacist should determine all agents that the patient is taking and, if appropriate, has taken in the past, including prescription drugs, nonprescription medications, physician samples, and herbal and nutritional agents. The dose, dosage form, route of administration, duration of therapy, and indication for each drug must also be obtained.

Most practitioners realize that patients may get prescriptions filled at several pharmacies, and therefore they inquire about medications obtained from all sources, including mail order. Patients may also borrow medications from family members or friends. Inquiries about medication sources must be made carefully so patients do not feel pressured to transfer all their prescriptions to a particular pharmacy.

Pharmacists also collect data on how patients take their medication at home. For example, if a medication is labeled to be taken three times per day, did the patient take the medication with meals, every 8 hours, or according to some other schedule? Pharmacists investigate the patient's compliance with therapy as well, asking questions in a nonjudgmental fashion. An example is, "People often find it difficult to remember to take all their medication. How often do you think you may forget to take a dose?" Storage conditions for medications should also be assessed.

The next step is to assess the patient's response to their medications using subjective and objective data. Asking questions that require patients to describe what the drug's effect has been generates a subjective response. (Drug effects may be either therapeutic or adverse.) Initial questions should generally be open-ended, such as, "How has your erythromycin been working for you?" The answers should allow the pharmacist to ask narrower follow-up questions, which may be closed-ended, such as, "Have you noticed any stomach upset from your erythromycin?"

Some drugs, such as cholesterol-lowering agents, do not have a readily identifiable subjective therapeutic response. In these cases, pharmacists must determine which objective data will allow them to assess therapeutic effect. Similarly, not all adverse effects will lead to subjective patient complaints, such as hyperglycemia caused by thiazides, so objective data may be required.

Medical History

Medical history, also known as disease-state history, is the other major grouping of information the pharmacist needs. It is difficult to assess if a patient is receiving the best medication when the pharmacist is uncertain of the disease being treated or the disease's status.

An adequate disease state history is more than a list. Using an appropriate mixture of open- and closed-ended questions, as well as subjective and objective data, the pharmacist must determine which disease states the patient is suffering from and which, if any, medications are being used to treat them.

Sometimes objective data may be generated in the pharmacy to assess the patient's disease states. Examples include vital signs, peak expiratory flow rates, blood sugars, serum lipid profiles, and coagulation parameters. Other data will have to come from the physician's office or hospital, and pharmacists will need to determine whether a release form is necessary.

In this portion of the information-gathering phase, the pharmacist may perform a modified review of systems (ROS), in which each organ system and the effect of drugs and diseases on that organ system, and vice versa, are reviewed. Pharmacists must learn how to focus their review and determine which organ systems must be evaluated and which may be safely ignored in a given patient.

An adequate disease state history is more than a list.

For example, inquiries about the vision of a diabetic are well advised, since diabetics commonly have visual problems. Patients with depression who are taking fluoxetine, which only rarely causes visual disturbances, might not require vision assessment. Pharmacists need to learn to modify a physician's review by asking the patient questions that provide information on an organ system's level of functioning. Some pharmacists find that this forces them to focus on what is both important and possible to accomplish in the community pharmacy setting.

Relevant subjective information includes patients' perceptions about which of their conditions have the greatest impact on quality of life. The pharmacist should also assess which diseases are currently stable, which are improving, and which are worsening. Finally, it is important to inquire how well patients understand their disease states and have insight into their care. Such information helps pharmacists prioritize when developing a care plan.

The Narrow History

At the end of a medication counseling session or when supplying a refill, pharmacists often find it useful to ask patients how well they think their medicines are working and if they have any questions, concerns, or problems. If the answer is "yes," the pharmacist can proceed with a narrowly focused data collection session based on the patient's responses. If the answer is "no," the pharmacist can proceed to the next patient. Given the time pressures that all pharmacists face, rapid screening methods such as these will ensure that patients get the care they need as efficiently as possible.

There is clear precedent in the health care system for using the narrow history. For example, if a physician sees a patient for the first time who complains of symptoms of a urinary tract infection, the physician will perform a work-up of the infection and only gather other data that could reasonably influence treatment selection, such as whether the patient has a history of diabetes or prostatic hyperplasia. If pharmacists are to be efficient care providers, they need to develop the same screening skills.

A narrowly focused initial screening interview can be useful not only to investigate and resolve a drug therapy problem, but also to help establish a therapeutic relationship with the patient. Later, the pharmacist will likely have the opportunity to offer the patient a more in-depth interview and complete the patient's history. Pharmacists may be uncomfortable making clinical decisions in the absence of complete information, but expanding a patient database by doing several short interviews over time is practical when a complete patient interview is impossible.

The Routine Care History

The Routine Care History is used as a means to choose which elements of a patient's history are essential to provide care for a suspected drug therapy problem. It requires the pharmacist to examine information that is readily available to him (patient profiles, demographic data, etc.) and use that information to collect a well-focused Narrow History. Pharmacists who are struggling with how to fit pharmaceutical care into a practice may find the Routine Care History a quick and efficient tool.

Although a lot of laboratory and other clinical information may not be readily available to community pharmacists, they do have quick and ready access to the following types of information: patient demographics; drug allergies; medication history; and a basic knowledge of pathophysiology and pharmacotherapy. Pharmacists using a Routine Care History have no more or better information than any other pharmacist; they just look at it differently and examine it more closely.

A narrowly focused initial screening interview can be useful not only to investigate and resolve a drug therapy problem, but also to help establish a therapeutic relationship with the patient. Later, the pharmacist will likely have the opportunity to offer the patient a more in-depth interview and complete the patient's history.

Demographic Information

By looking at patient demographic information a bit differently, pharmacists can determine if the patient has unusually high risks for a drug therapy problem. If so, they can use the information to perform a Narrow History.

Extremes of age (i.e., the very young and the very old) is an example of demographic data that pharmacists should consider. When filling a prescription and performing the usual drug utilization review (DUR) required by law in many states, a pharmacist can ask herself what effect the patient's age could have on the following issues:

• Drug selection.

• Dose selection.

• Kidney and liver function.

• The effect of cognitive impairments or development on compliance.

• The effect of manual dexterity or visual impairment on drug taking.

For example, a pharmacist is filling an antibiotic prescription for a 2-year-old child with an ear infection. Simple knowledge of the patient's age should direct the pharmacist to consider the following:

• Is this the right dose for the patient's age and weight?

• Who will be administering the drug to the child: a parent, a day care provider, or both? Does the caregiver have a measuring device to administer an accurate dose?

• Will storage of the medication be an issue if the child travels between home and day care?

Having asked herself these questions, the pharmacist can gather information to determine if there is a risk for a dosage, compliance, or drug stability-related problems. Adequate attention to demographic matters can prevent some drug therapy problems from occurring.

Other demographic information pharmacists can consider would include the effects of a patient's living conditions, income, and job on compliance, medication use, and medication storage.

Allergies

Using allergy information extends beyond recording that the patient is allergic to penicillin. Pharmacists should also consider the following:

• Does the medication history suggest any current medications are being used to treat an allergy problem (e.g., long-term steroids, antihistamines)?

• What is the allergic potential of the patient's drug regimen?

• Is there any evidence to suggest the patient may benefit from prophylactic therapy (e.g., epinephrine pen, antihistamines)?

If the assessment of the patient's allergy information suggests there is the potential for a drug therapy problem, a Narrow History can be used for evaluation.

Medication History

Ideally, the pharmacist will know the patient's complete drug history including nonprescription medications, samples, herbal and nutritional supplements, and prescriptions filled elsewhere. However, if the only medication history available is on the dispensing computer, application of Routine Care History techniques can still provide valuable, if possibly incomplete, opportunities for the pharmacist to provide pharmaceutical care.

The pharmacist must think critically about the information she has. She must try to decide if anything in the patient's profile suggests that medication needs are not being met. Drug therapy problems developing from unmet needs in the area of the indication for drug therapy are "unnecessary drug therapy" and "needs additional drug therapy."

Every drug must have an appropriate indication, and every indication that requires drug therapy should receive such therapy. The Routine Medication History requires the pharmacist to evaluate by asking the following questions:

• Is there any evidence of duplicate therapy?

• Is any combination therapy clinically rational?

• Are those conditions that typically require combination therapy being treated in that manner?

- Is the patient taking any nonprescription medication for the same indication as any of his prescription drugs?

- Is the patient taking any medication on a long-term basis for conditions that are generally self-limited?

- Is any long-term use of hypnotics, anxiolytics, or analgesics clinically rational?

- Are any of the medications being used to treat an adverse effect caused by another medication?

Drug therapy problems related to unmet needs for effectiveness are "wrong drug" and "dosage too low." Assessing risks for these problems may be done by asking the following questions:

- Are there frequent changes in drug therapy, dose, dosage schedule, or other aspects of the medication regimen?

- Is the patient taking any nonprescription medications for the same condition as a prescription drug?

- Is the medication selected optimal for its indication?

- Does the condition generally respond well to this drug therapy?

- Does the drug have any special storage or administration requirements the patient may have difficulty with?

- Is there a need for combination or additional therapy?

- Are the dose, dosage form, and dosage interval appropriate?

- Can the patient's organ systems have any effect on drug effectiveness?

- What are the possible drug interactions and is there any evidence of them?

- What are the possible adverse drug reactions and is there any evidence of them?

The answers to these questions will direct the pharmacist to the sort of information that needs to be gathered during a Narrow History.

Drug therapy problems that are related to the patient's need for safety are "adverse drug reactions" and "dosage too high." The patient's risk for such problems can be assessed with the following screening questions:

• What is the adverse effect and drug interaction profile of each drug?

• What is the effect of the patient's organ systems on each drug and what is the effect of each drug on the patient's organ systems?

• Are the dose, dosage interval, and duration of therapy reasonable—especially in light of the patient's likely renal and hepatic function?

• Is the dose being increased/decreased too quickly/slowly?

• Is this drug the safest one for this condition?

• Can the patient self administer this drug correctly?

Finally, compliance can be assessed by considering the following questions:

• Are the refill dates and quantities consistent with correct medication use?

• Is the drug regimen so complex as to influence compliance?

• Could the number of doses to be taken each day influence compliance?

• Does the patient have a history of obtaining only a partial fill of a prescription?

• How often does the patient need to come to the pharmacy to refill a prescription?

Communicating with Patients

Communications that all pharmacists engage in daily include patient counseling, recommending nonprescription therapy, answering patient drug information questions, and similar activities. Like patient medication profiles, when coupled with Routine Care History techniques these communication episodes are resources that can be used to provide more effective patient care.

During interactions such as patient counseling or recommending nonprescription medication, etc., information generally flows from the pharmacist to the patient. In these situations, the pharmacist delivers factual information the patient needs to learn. Using routine patient care techniques, the pharmacist turns these communication situations into a two-way flow of information to see if any additional Narrow History can be gathered to assess the patient.

Here is an actual example observed in a community pharmacy. A patient approached the pharmacist and asked, "Bill, can Prinivil cause a cough?" The pharmacist replied that it could. The patient then left the pharmacy, apparently satisfied with the answer, and the pharmacist went back to work believing he had answered the question.

The pharmacist could have turned the exchange into a two-way communication by recognizing that something beyond simple curiosity about a drug's side effect profile was behind the question. He could have added, "Medications can have a wide variety of side effects. If you have noticed a cough recently, please tell me about it." This type of communication could have helped the pharmacist recognize a drug therapy problem.

Self Assessment Questions

3.1 Are the following examples of subjective or objective information? Justify your answer.

a. During an interview, a patient tells you he takes his blood pressure medication correctly five or six days a week.

b. While doing a pill count as a compliance check, you determine that 30 blood pressure tablets with instructions to take one tablet daily have lasted the patient 36 days.

c. The nursing staff in the aged care facility check off each dose administered in the patient's medication administration record (MAR). For the month of April, there is a check mark daily for each blood pressure tablet given, which indicates 100% compliance.

d. According to your computer, your patient gets his monthly blood pressure medications refilled every 33 days.

3.2 How should the pharmacists in the following cases begin developing therapeutic relationships?

a. Jeanette Tepperman appears to be in her mid 50s. She presents pharmacist Ryan White with a new prescription for conjugated estrogens 0.625 mg tablets Sig: 1 tablet qd x 30 refill x 3.
When Ryan scans her profile, he sees she has never had this medication, or progesterone, before. Ryan knows that women with an intact uterus who take estrogens unopposed by progesterone are at higher risk for uterine cancer. To determine Mrs. Tepperman's risk for a drug therapy problem (adverse drug reaction causing uterine cancer) Ryan must ask if she has had a hysterectomy.

b. Melanie Frith, a clinical pharmacist on the cardiology service, is performing a history on Lionel Wilkens, a man in his 40s who is being evaluated for new onset angina. He is vague when describing the circumstances in which the angina occurred. Mr. Watson has a slight flush to his face that Melanie recognizes as common in men of his age who have taken sildenafil or a similar agent for erectile dysfunction. Mr. Wilkens may have to start taking nitrate medications for his chest pain and nitrates are contra-indicated with sildenafil.

3.3 How can a pharmacist use the characteristics below to qualify patients for pharmaceutical care?

a. Patients who receive frequent refills of albuterol inhalers from community pharmacists.

b. Patients who are frequently admitted to the hospital with recurrent episodes of congestive heart failure and pulmonary edema.

c. Nursing home patients receiving more than five scheduled medications per day.

3.4 Reword the following into well worded, open-ended questions.

a. Do your iron tablets make you constipated?

b. Did you have to take several nitroglycerin pills to get relief?

c. Do you have any other questions about your diabetes medication?

d. Will you remember to take your blood pressure medicine as the doctor has instructed?

e. Are you getting prescriptions filled at any other pharmacies?

3.5 Compare the Basic Seven questions with the three Public Health Service questions. In which patient situations do they work best? How well do the questions uncover drug therapy problems related to compliance, adverse effects, and need for additional drug therapy?

3.6 Reword the following without using pharmacists' jargon.

a. What was your diastolic pressure in the doctor's office?

b. What is your renal and hepatic function like?

c. How severe is the neuropathy from your didanosine?

d. Is there a history of coronary artery disease in your family?

3.7 In the following case, how might the pharmacist interpret these responses?

On the form in Figure 3-1 a patient has included the following agents under Prescription Medication History: Albuterol Inhaler, 2 puffs qid prn; Fluticasone Inhaler 44 microgram, 2 puffs bid; prednisone 5 mg tablets 40 mg burst then taper as required for asthma flare; doxycyline 100 mg po qd x 7 days when sputum color changes or febrile.

The patient has answered "Yes" to the following questions: abdominal pain or cramps; frequent heartburn/indigestion; shortness of breath.

3.8 Which of the following items should be included in every history taken by a pharmacist and which need not be included?

a. Complete medication history including samples and non-prescription medications.

b. Caffeine intake.

c. Family history.

d. Medication compliance.

e. Height and weight.

3.9 What subjective or objective information would you collect to assess the patient's response (both clinical and adverse) to the following medications?

a. Esomeprazole taken for gastro-esophageal reflux disease (GERD).

b. Sertraline taken for depression.

c. Glipizide taken for Type 2 diabetes.

3.10 Consider the following patient profile. How can the pharmacist use a Routine Care History to evaluate the patient's risk for a drug therapy problem?

Name: Viola Devlin   Address: 1324 McAllen Blvd   Date of Birth 11/4/1924

Date	Drug/Strength	Sig	Qty	Refills
Feb 20	Altace 2.5 mg	1 qd	30	6
Feb 27	Furosemide 20 mg	1 qd	30	6
Feb 27	Digoxin 0.25 mg	1 qd	30	2
Mar 6	Synthroid 0.1 mg	1 qd	30	2

3.11 Consider the following patient profile. How can the pharmacist use a Routine Care History to evaluate this patient's risk for a drug therapy problem?

Name: Miranda Ortiz   Address: 543 Wilson Crt   Date of Birth 1/24/1942

Date	Drug/Strength	Sig	Qty	Refills
Feb 20	Xalatan	1 qtt out qhs	2.5mL	6
Feb 27	Regular Insulin	8u ac bkfast/supper	10mL	6
Feb 27	NPH Insulin	16u ac bkfast	10mL	6

3.12 Consider the following patient profile. How can the pharmacist use a Routine Care History to evaluate this patient's risk for a drug therapy problem?

Name: Ken Rizzuto   Address: 870 Flagler Rd   Date of Birth 12/2/1972
Ken presents new prescriptions for Lariam Tablets x 6 Sig 1 weekly; Levaquin 500 mg x 3 Sig 1 po qd prn diarrhea and Lomotil x 12 Sig 1 prn diarrhea.

Date	Drug/Strength	Sig	Qty	Refills
Feb 27	Humulin 70/30	8u ac meals	10mL	6

3.13 A patient asks, "Does Dilantin go into my breast milk?" How can the pharmacist's response promote a two-way communication that can help identify any drug therapy problems?

Reflection Question

Think about a pharmacy that you have seen or worked in. What areas in the pharmacy could be used for a consultation area? What types of minor changes would have to occur to provide a suitable space?

References

1. Boyce RW, Herrier RN. Obtaining and using patient data. *Am Pharm.* 1991;NS31:517–23.

2. de Bittner MR, Michocki R. Establishing a pharmaceutical care database. *J Am Pharm Assoc.* 1996;NS36:60-9.

3. Bell DL. HIPAA update. *J Am Pharm Assoc.* 2002;58(5):8-11, 36.

Patient Data Evaluation

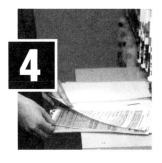

4

John P. Rovers

fter interviewing the patient and collecting subjective and objective information, the pharmacist is still at the entry point to the Pharmaceutical Care Cycle illustrated in Chapter 2. What must be done now is to assess the information to determine whether the patient is, in fact, suffering from drug therapy problems. When drug therapy problems are identified, the patient truly enters the Pharmaceutical Care Cycle. This chapter reviews in detail how to evaluate patients and their drug therapy.

Systematic Approach Is Key

It is best to use a systematic, reproducible method for data evaluation similar to that used for data collection. Other professions use this method. When a dentist examines a patient's mouth, for example, he will start his examination on the same tooth each time so he is not missing problems or identifying them incorrectly. Similarly, if pharmacists evaluate all patient information in the same organized, systematic fashion each time, they will be much more successful at identifying all the patient's drug therapy problems.

To a practitioner who is just beginning the transformation into a pharmaceutical care provider, the number of steps and concepts presented here may appear daunting. The good news is that drug therapy evaluation is not nearly as complicated as it seems initially. In this chapter, the beginner is walked through the process step by step.

Very few patients need to have all these issues evaluated every time, so experts learn to edit the process and eventually it becomes automatic. The most time-consuming part is often updating knowledge about a drug or a disease.

As pharmacists gain experience, data gathering and data evaluation steps come to occur almost simultaneously. While pharmacists are accumulating facts from the patient interview, they as-

In this chapter, the following concepts are reviewed:

- Evaluating a patient's history in a systematic fashion.

- Evaluating if a patient's drug-related needs are being met.

- Evaluating if medication is safe and effective.

- Identifying poor medication compliance and identifying causes of compliance problems.

- Identifying drug therapy problems by determining how to fix them.

sess the information and identify drug therapy problems. For experts the processes of gathering the patient's history (Chapter 3), assessing the history to identify any drug therapy problems (Chapter 4), and devising a care plan (Chapter 5) are seamless. Practice results in increased speed and better clinical skills.

In Chapter 2, it was noted that drug therapy problems are derived from five patient needs for drug therapy: appropriate indication, effectiveness, safety, compliance, and untreated indications. Evaluating these needs and ensuring that they are met is the basis of the pharmacist's assessment.

Following a systematic method, pharmacists are able to pinpoint actual drug therapy problems, identify potential problems, or discover if they must gather more information. Most practitioners do not merely use a series of standardized questions. Instead they focus on the patient's drugs and diseases as a way to assess needs and identify problems. See Table 2-4, page 33 for a listing of the drug therapy problems associated with specific drug-related needs.

The self assessment exercises in this chapter will help with practicing each step in data analysis. Applying the principles discussed in each section of this chapter to data obtained from an actual patient is a good way to become familiar with the process.

TABLE 4-1

Case Study

Mrs. Annette Rikfin is a 75-year-old patient of Dr. Renée Hale. On June 26/ this year Dr. Hale asks ambulatory care clinic pharmacist David Rice to perform a full medication evaluation on Mrs. Rifkin and report back his findings and recommendations. After interviewing the patient and gathering a complete medication history (as described in Chapter 3), David then verifies as much information as possible from the patient's clinic chart and from the clinic's dispensing computer. A summary of the patient's information obtained from all sources is below:

History supplied by Mrs. Rifkin:

Medication	Dose per patient	Indication per patient
Calcium Carbonate (OTC)	1500 mg qd	brittle bones
EC ASA (OTC)	81 mg qd	thin blood
Esomeprazole	40 mg qd	heartburn
Nitroglycerin spray 400mcg	1–2 sprays as needed	chest pain
Amlodipine	5 mg qd	blood pressure

A PRACTICAL GUIDE TO PHARMACEUTICAL CARE: A Clinical Skills Primer

TABLE 4-1

History supplied by Mrs. Rifkin: continued

Medication	Dose per patient	Indication per patient
Acetaminophen w Codeine 30mg	1 tablet prn (uses 1–2/week)	foot/knee pain
Tiotropium capsules for inhalation	18 mcg by inhalation qd	asthma
Atenolol	50 mg qd	blood pressure
Nitroglycerin Patch	0.2 mg/hr patch qd	chest pain
Ramipril	10 mg qd	blood pressure
Acetaminophen (OTC)	1g q4h (takes once a week)	pain

Patient comments: Mrs. Rifkin claims to not have any problems taking her medications and says she usually misses only a few pills per month. She has no difficulty using her nitroglycerin spray or patch nor the tiotropium capsules for inhalation. Her major complaint at this point is fatigue that starts shortly after she arises each morning and begins to resolve by mid-to-late afternoon. Other than the fatigue, Mrs. Rifkin believes she is in good health and overall, says she feels well.

History from patient chart:

Drug Allergies: Irbesartan, celecoxib, doxycycline, simvastatin.

Current medical conditions: angina, Type 2 diabetes (diet controlled); gastro-esophageal reflux disease (GERD); hypertension; osteoarthritis with right total knee replacement.

Physical Exam: BP 130/70 Weight 169 pounds (77 kg), remaining vitals signs normal.

Most Recent Laboratory Results: sodium 141 mEq/L, potassium 4.4 mEq/L, chloride 106 mEq/L, bicarbonate 26 mEq/L, blood urea nitrogen 18 mg/dL, creatinine 0.7 mg/dL, blood glucose 96 mg/dL, glycosylated hemoglobin 6.5%, hemoglobin 14.2 g/L, hematocrit 38%, white blood cells 3,400 (normal differential), platelets 150,000, total cholesterol 205 mg/dL, triglycerides 142 mg/dL, HDL cholesterol 44 mg/dl, LDL cholesterol 133mg/dl.

Vaccination History: influenza and pneumococcal vaccines up to date.

Social History: widowed, lives alone in own home, good health and prescription drug insurance, non-smoker, occasional alcohol use.

History from Dispensing Computer:

Medication list identical to that provided by patient except computer does not show nonpresciption calcium carbonate, EC ASA, and acetaminophen. Checking the dispensing computer pharmacist David Rice notes the following:

Medication	Sig	Quantity	Last Refilled
Esomeprazole 40 mg	1 qd	30	June 6/this year
Nitroglycerin spray 400 mcg	2 sprays prn	1 unit	December 8/last year
Amlodipine 5 mg	1 qd	30	June 11/this year
Acetaminophen w Codeine 30 mg	1–2 bid	100	August 20/last year
Tiotropium Inhaler Capsules	1 qd	30	June 11/this year
Atenolol 50 mg	1 qd	30	June 19/this year
Nitroglycerin Patch 0.2 mg/hr	1 qd	30	June 21/this year
Ramipril 10 mg	1 qd	30	June 11/this year

Comparing Problems and Treatments

After determining a patient's medical conditions, symptoms, and drug therapies, the pharmacist must compare the patient's medical problems and medication list. The pharmacist needs to answer these questions:

• Are all conditions being managed?

• Are all drug therapies managing a condition?

The answer to these questions will determine whether two of the patient's needs for drug therapy ("no untreated indications" and "an indication for each drug") are being met.

The fastest and easiest way to begin this step is with a rapid screening. Pharmacists should prepare a list of all the drugs a patient is taking. Then they place a list of all of the patient's diseases, signs, symptoms, clinical complaints, etc., next to the first list. The pharmacist can then compare the information on the two lists by drawing a line connecting each drug to its related disease or symptom. If there are drugs, clinical complaints, diseases, etc., that are not connected to another item, this may be the place to begin a detailed assessment.

A more rigorous methodology is likely to result in a more thorough patient evaluation. First, the pharmacist determines what is being done to manage medical conditions and symptoms. The patient may be taking one or more medications for each condition, and some conditions are managed by methods other than drug therapy.

Common nondrug therapies are diet, exercise, and surgery. Diet and exercise are therapeutic mainstays for patients with diabetes, hypertension, and other chronic conditions. An additional nondrug therapy, known as "watchful waiting," is a form of intensive patient monitoring. Physicians commonly use it when the benefits of starting drug therapy may not outweigh the risks. Patients with certain cardiac dysrhythmias, such as premature ventricular contractions, or patients who may be developing hypertension are frequently managed this way.

Until the disease is severe enough to place the patient at risk, the physician may simply elect to re-evaluate the patient at frequent intervals. The intention of "watchful waiting" is to carefully monitor the patient and only institute therapy when it is clearly indicated. Pharmacists should not confuse "watchful waiting" with doing nothing. Doing nothing suggests drug therapy is unlikely to be indicated, ever.

Untreated Indications

If the pharmacist establishes that a disease is not being managed by either drug or nondrug therapy, she can conclude that the patient's need related to "untreated indications" is not being met. But if one or more symptoms are not being treated, she cannot necessarily conclude that the patient has a drug therapy problem. Only after the symptom has been evaluated, and is determined not to have been caused by a drug, can the pharmacist safely say that additional therapy may be needed.

If the patient has an untreated indication, the pharmacist must discover why. Sometimes the patient has never sought medical attention. In these cases, the pharmacist is qualified to observe that the patient exhibits signs or symptoms consistent with a disease state which merit medical evaluation, and that those signs or symptoms are generally managed with drug therapy. When presenting observations to a physician, the pharmacist can say, "I am referring the patient back to you for medical evaluation." This makes it clear that he is not making a diagnosis.

Another cause for an untreated condition is a need for synergistic or prophylactic therapy. Patients with hypertension or an infection, for example, may need synergistic therapy to supplement the therapy already being administered. A patient with atrial fibrillation who is not being treated with an anticoagulant may need prophylactic therapy to prevent blood clots.

TABLE 4-2

Questions to Consider

- Is there an untreated indication? Why?

- Does the patient need synergistic therapy to supplement therapy already being administered?

- Does the patient need prophylactic therapy?

- Does each medication the patient is taking correlate with a medical condition?

- Is the patient misusing medication, whether unintentionally or deliberately?

- Would nondrug therapy be preferable for any of the patient's conditions?

- Is the patient taking duplicate therapy without adequate cause?

- Are any drugs being administered unnecessarily to treat adverse effects?

Indication for Each Drug

Once the pharmacist is satisfied that each condition is being treated (appropriateness of treatment will be considered later), the next step is to ensure that each medication correlates with a medical condition. If the pharmacist cannot state with certainty why a patient is taking a medication, the drug therapy may not be necessary. But he should also think about whether more data are needed. Sometimes patients do not know the indication for their medications.

Sometimes the status of a medical condition changes without a commensurate change in drug therapy. Patients who were started on medication for an acute condition while they were in the hospital are particularly at risk. The continuity of care between the hospital and ambulatory settings is often problematic, and confusions with medications are common. Pharmacists trained in pharmaceutical care practice have reported cases where patients received laxatives or nitrates for many years after hospital discharge, even if their conditions were resolved. The patients simply assumed that the doctor wanted them to continue; the doctor simply assumed that the patient was chronically constipated or had ongoing angina.

Patients may misuse their medications unintentionally, but they may also misuse them deliberately. Most pharmacists are already attuned to inappropriate drug-seeking behavior by patients. Because pharmaceutical care practitioners have a greater patient database available, they can verify indications for drug therapy and reach conclusions about misuse more confidently.

As pharmacists ensure that each drug has an appropriate indication, they should also determine if nondrug therapy would be preferable. Nonprescription medications are more likely to be used unnecessarily than prescription ones. When patients attempt self-care, they typically do not try to balance the risks and benefits of drug versus nondrug therapy. For example, patients frequently take vitamins for "energy," a use for which they are ineffective. A pharmaceutical care provider can work with a patient to review diet, exercise, and sleep patterns and institute a nondrug therapeutic plan.

Taking duplicate therapy without adequate cause is also a drug therapy problem. In the past, such problems were typically identified by computer screening programs. Since these programs do not use patient-specific data, some problems turned out to be a deliberate, rational use of two medications. Using a pharma-

TABLE 4-3

Common Nondrug Therapies

- Diet.

- Exercise.

- Surgery.

- "Watchful waiting": intensive patient monitoring.

A PRACTICAL GUIDE TO PHARMACEUTICAL CARE: A Clinical Skills Primer

ceutical care model, the pharmacist is able to determine whether duplicate therapy is rational pharmacotherapy.

The final problem related to appropriateness of indication is using a drug unnecessarily to treat the adverse effects of a second drug. Patients who are on multiple medications (the elderly are often at particular risk) may have this problem. Some pharmacists use a 10:1 rule of thumb: that is, for every 10 medications a patient is taking, one of them is to treat a side effect of one of the other nine. If the patient does not need the medication causing the adverse effect, or if it can be safely changed to another medication without the same side-effect profile, then clearly it is a case of an avoidable adverse effect. If, on the other hand, the drug causing the adverse effect cannot be changed or discontinued, then the adverse effect is unavoidable and may need to be treated.

So far in the patient work-up, the pharmacist has ensured that every medication has an indication and that every indication has a medication (or at least a therapy). The pharmacist is now able to assess whether the patient's needs of "appropriate indication" and "untreated indication" have been met. Furthermore, the pharmacist should be able to identify any drug therapy problems related to these needs. If the pharmacist still cannot make this assessment confidently, then he needs to gather further data and repeat the evaluation.

Safety, Efficacy, and Compliance

Drug therapy problems related to safety and efficacy are among the most common areas for pharmacist–physician conflict. To manage these discussions the pharmacist needs to have adequate evidence from patient-specific data showing that the patient demonstrates, or is at risk for, harm from the drug therapy problem.

Consider the following example: A pharmacist is about to refill a prescription for digoxin 0.25 mg, to be taken by mouth once a day, for a 77-year-old man who is transferring his prescription into the pharmacy. Using the old model of practice, the pharmacist might determine that the patient's potential drug therapy problem would be "dosage too high." In a phone call to the physician all he can do is voice his concern that, according to the literature, 0.25 mg of digoxin is a high dose in elderly patients, who often have some renal impairment. Under a pharmaceutical care model, however, the pharmacist would have gathered patient-specific data such as pulse rate. If the patient demonstrated bradycardia, the pharmacist would have much stronger information to back up his claim of excessive dosage.

Drug therapy problems related to safety and efficacy are among the most common areas for pharmacist–physician conflict.

When pharmacists evaluate pharmacotherapy for drug therapy problems related to safety and efficacy, they must try to use patient-specific information as often as possible. Otherwise, they are less likely to convince physicians that a problem exists.

Unlike patient needs related to indication, it is difficult to evaluate needs related to safety, efficacy, and compliance one at a time. The evaluation can still be done systematically, but the same question may cover more than one patient need.

To draw valid conclusions, the pharmacist must follow an organized approach and use as much patient-specific information as possible. First the pharmacist must review the dose, dosage interval, duration of therapy, and dosage form for each drug on the patient's medication list. Since this practice requires the pharmacist to review both the drugs themselves and the patient's response to them, it provides evidence of how well the patient's drug needs for safety and efficacy are being met.

Appropriateness of the Dose

Is each drug's dose appropriate, too high, or too low? This is the first question pharmacists should ask themselves during their systematic evaluation. Judgments on the appropriateness of the medication strength should be made using patient-specific data such as age, weight, concurrent drugs and diseases, pregnancy or lactation status, and so on. It is best not to depend solely on the dosing information in a reference text, unless absolutely necessary.

To definitively evaluate the appropriateness of the dose, it is necessary to assess the patient's response to the medication. If a dose is felt to be too low but subjective and/or objective data suggest that the patient is responding to the drug, it is difficult to justify a conclusion that the patient has an actual drug therapy problem of too low a dose. Similarly, if a patient does not exhibit signs or symptoms of adverse effects or toxicity, concluding that there is an actual problem of too high a dose may not be plausible. This does not guarantee that there is no potential drug therapy problem here, only that the evidence for the existence of a problem seems weak.

Yet potential drug therapy problems are often identified by determining a patient's risk using information from the literature. For example, a patient with impaired renal function is receiving a "normal" dose of lithium carbonate for his mania. Lithium is a potentially toxic drug excreted by the kidneys. A drug information handbook suggests that the dose of lithium should be decreased by 25% to 75%, depending on the patient's kidney function. Even if this patient does not exhibit the sedation or confusion normally seen with lithium toxicity, the patient does have a potential drug therapy problem because the risks and consequences of lithium toxicity are severe.

A final thing to consider when evaluating dose is how long the patient has been taking it. As renal or hepatic function decreases with age, drug dose is often decreased. Sometimes this does not happen and the patient gradually develops toxic drug levels. In summary, evidence of clinical response, evidence of adverse effects, and potential risk for harm should all be considered when evaluating the appropriateness of the patient's dose.

Once the appropriate strength of the patient's medication has been prescribed, the pharmacist can move on to consider other reasons why the dose may not be optimal. When patients store medications in an excessively hot and humid location, or if the medication is past its expiration date, the dosage form may degrade enough that the patient receives a subtherapeutic dose. Similarly, when patients administer their medication incorrectly, they may receive too high or too low a dose, even if the initial choice of dose was well made. Finally, the pharmacist should screen for any drug interactions that may result in potential or actual exposure to toxic or subtherapeutic drug levels. If no clinical evidence of a drug interaction is present, then the pharmacist should assess how likely the emergence of the interaction is and how severe its consequences may be.

TABLE 4-4

Questions to Consider

• Are the dose, dosage interval, duration of therapy, and dosage form appropriate for each medication the patient is taking?

• How long has the patient been receiving the current dose of each medication?

• Is the patient responding appropriately to the drug?

• Is there evidence of adverse effects or drug allergies?

• Are the medications being stored properly and are any past their expiration dates?

• Are medications being administered correctly?

• Are there any potential or actual drug interactions?

Dosage Schedule

Is the dosage schedule appropriate, too frequent, or too infrequent? This question is related both to the patient's need for safe and efficacious drug therapy and to whether a dosage is too high or too low.

Dosage interval is evaluated in the same fashion as dosage strength; the patient's clinical response and evidence of toxicity must be examined. If no sign of undesirable outcomes is found, the patient does not have an actual drug therapy problem. There may still be a potential problem which would be pinpointed in the same way as potential problems related to dosage strength.

Duration of Therapy

Is the duration of each drug therapy appropriate, too long, or too short? The same issues apply as for dosage strength and interval. Patient-specific data must be evaluated, if possible, before the pharmacist concludes that an actual problem exists, and literature may be used to justify the existence of a potential problem.

Dosage Form

No other health care provider has the training in dosage forms that pharmacists have. Pharmaceutical care providers put this knowledge to use by evaluating the appropriateness of each dosage form for their patients.

Problems with dosage form seem to be found most commonly with inhaled medications, which the pharmacist identifies by checking a patient's technique with a metered dose or other inhaler. However, there are issues with other routes of administration. Injection technique and appropriateness of the parenteral route should be evaluated for patients' self-injecting medications while at home.

Depending on the dosage form being considered, pharmacists should ask themselves a variety of questions:

- Does the patient have the visual acuity and manual dexterity to prepare a dose accurately?

- Will a topical, otic, ophthalmic, or rectal dosage form be stored and administered correctly?

- Do the patient's job or school activities prevent him from using the dosage form properly?

No other health care provider has the training in dosage forms that pharmacists have.

- If the patient is using a patch, does she understand how to apply it and how often to change it?

- Can the patient physically swallow all oral dosage forms or is he crushing them?

- Are sustained-release products being used correctly?

- Are liquid dosage forms measured accurately before being administered? Are they stored correctly and shaken before use as required?

- Are sublingual products being used correctly?

The Right or Wrong Drug

After evaluating the dosage form, the pharmacist must ensure that each drug the patient is taking is the right one for the condition. Arguments of "right drug" versus "wrong drug" are as old as clinical pharmacy and have historically been a significant area of tension between pharmacists and physicians. Declaring that a patient suffers from the problem of "wrong drug" can inadvertently offend a physician. Since the pharmacist–physician relationship often plays an important role in how problems related to drug therapy choice are evaluated and solved, being aware of the different perspectives of professionals is essential. Historically, the physician's primary consideration was the patient, while for the pharmacist, it was usually the drug therapy or maybe the prescription.

In addition, pharmacists and physicians tend to use different data to make decisions. Physicians use a combination of what they know from their reading and what they have learned from managing similar patients in the past. Since most pharmacists have historically neither managed nor monitored patients in any significant sense, they tend to base their decisions on what they have read, rather than on what they have done.

TABLE 4-5

Questions to Consider

- Is each drug the patient takes the right one for the condition?
- Does the patient have any clear contraindications to a drug?
- Is the patient's condition refractory to the therapy?
- Is more effective therapy available than the agent that the patient is on?

The task of pharmaceutical care providers is to change this situation and demonstrate that the patient is at the center of their efforts. This is best accomplished by having a solid grasp of the patient-specific facts, a good knowledge base of drugs and diseases, and, perhaps most important, an open mind. Disagreements sometimes derive from physicians not realizing what motivates pharmacists. Pharmacists need to help physicians understand that patient care is their mutual, primary interest.

The issue of a wrong drug caused by an inappropriate dosage form is an example of a drug therapy problem for which the physician is more disposed to accept the pharmacist's judgment.

Contraindications

If a patient has a clear contraindication to a drug, there is a problem with wrong choice of drug. Physicians are generally inclined to accept pharmacists' recommendations in such cases because choosing a clearly contraindicated drug opens them up to a lawsuit. Often, however, the contraindication is relative, not absolute.

For example, a woman may have osteoporosis but also require therapy with prednisone for her systemic lupus erythematosus. Since steroids may exacerbate her osteoporosis, they would be relatively contraindicated in such a patient unless the possible benefits of the steroids are greater than the risks.

Making that determination is a possible source of conflict between physicians and pharmacists. Relative contraindications are a matter of judgment, and the pharmacist and physician will not always agree on how important a relative contraindication is. Patient-specific data and a good knowledge of the literature are the pharmacist's key tools for dealing with questions of possible contraindications.

Refractory Conditions or More Effective Therapy

Another reason for deciding a drug is wrong is that the patient's condition is refractory to the therapy. This may be seen, for example, in patients on oral hypoglycemic therapy who have not responded to maximal doses of multiple drugs. In patients whose diabetes may have become refractory to sulfonylureas, the role of insulin or insulin sensitizers needs to be explored.

In addition, the patient may not be responding to therapy because the drug being used is not indicated for the condition, or there may be more effective drug therapy available. These are all judgment calls. Whether a condition has become refractory

A PRACTICAL GUIDE TO PHARMACEUTICAL CARE: A Clinical Skills Primer

can only be determined if there is convincing evidence, either subjective or objective, that the patient is no longer responding to therapy. Because this conclusion involves decisions about pathophysiology and how the disease state is progressing, physicians may view pharmacists' involvement as an attempt to diagnose or evaluate a disease state.

The question of whether a more effective therapy is available to treat a condition is a common source of interprofessional conflict. If a physician has had good clinical success with a given drug in a certain situation, the pharmacist may find it difficult to convince him that it is a poor therapeutic choice. And sometimes physicians select a certain drug because it is new and they want to try it in a few patients.

The drug therapy problem of "wrong drug" can cause difficulty for beginning pharmaceutical care practitioners. Pharmacists may feel apprehensive since the problems appear to be so controversial. But keep in mind that physicians can and do make errors in choosing medications. When they do, they are generally receptive to the pharmacist's opinions, especially when the opinions are phrased in a way that reflects the pharmacist's concern for the patient.

Rational decisions on the choice of drug therapy, as well as choices related to dose, dosage intervals, and duration of therapy, reflect both the art and science of pharmacotherapeutic decision-making. Pharmacists must realize that competent, well-intentioned professionals can and do disagree. Much of the time they have reached different conclusions from the same data.

BOX 4-1

Unapproved Indications

"Indication" refers to more than the federally approved indications listed in the product monograph. Physicians sometimes use drugs for nonindicated conditions, most often because they have read medical literature that supports the drug's usefulness in treating the condition. Although the drug is not officially approved for a certain use, they have evidence that it may be effective, and prescribe accordingly. In other instances, physicians combine what they know of the patient's pathophysiology and the drug's pharmacology to make a considered decision that the drug is likely to be effective.

Before pharmacists conclude that a drug is not indicated they should determine if there is at least a theoretical reason why the drug could work. If not, the pharmacist needs to find out if the physician is aware of information with which the pharmacist is not familiar.

Identifying a compliance problem is only the first step. Pharmacists must also discover the cause of the patient's noncompliance and consider a variety of possible solutions to the problem.

Pharmaceutical care providers learn not to be emotionally overinvested in these types of disagreements. They take them in stride and learn from them. They work hard to keep the lines of communication with the physician open so that, as less arguable problems are discovered, the physician will be receptive to the pharmacist's input.

Compliance Issues

Next, the pharmacist addresses the patient's need for compliance with drug therapy. Most pharmacists have spent their careers assisting patients with compliance problems. Unfortunately, a pharmacist faced with a noncompliant patient typically only provides additional counseling. In a pharmaceutical care practice, however, identifying a compliance problem is only the first step; pharmacists must also discover the cause of the patient's noncompliance and consider a wider variety of possible solutions to the problem.

Typically, pharmacists detect noncompliance by checking refill dates or performing actual pill counts. Pharmaceutical care practitioners will also use the patient interview as an opportunity to ask how the patient has complied with drug therapy. Most causes of inappropriate compliance can only be identified by evaluating the information gathered in the patient interview.

Occasionally, a patient cannot be compliant because the drug product is not available. It may be a new drug that is not yet in the wholesaler's catalogue, it may have been discontinued, or it may be back-ordered by the manufacturer. In these cases, the pharmacist will need to work with the physician and patient to find alternative therapy.

Sometimes patients exhibit poor compliance because they cannot afford the cost of the drug therapy. Most pharmacists are familiar with this situation and will try, when possible, to

---

TABLE 4-6

Questions to Consider

- Is the patient complying with drug therapy, and if not, why not?
- If the patient finds a therapy too expensive, what alternatives are possible?
- What are the possible disadvantages to switching therapy?

---

switch the patient to a more affordable agent. Although this situation does represent an actual drug therapy problem, the pharmacist must carefully consider the possible disadvantages of switching therapies when developing the care plan (see Chapter 5).

Changing drugs on the basis of cost alone is not always wise. In a patient whose disease is stable and who is not exhibiting problems with adverse effects or drug interactions, changing to another agent may place the patient at risk for new problems (including loss of clinical efficacy or side effects). Patients often cite cost as a plausible cause of poor compliance (even when such compliance is not truly related to cost). Sometimes when the patient perceives a drug cost as excessive, patient education on the nature of costs versus benefits is all that is required to remedy a compliance problem.

An inability to swallow or otherwise administer the dosage form is another cause for inappropriate compliance. Generally, pharmacists will identify this problem when they evaluate the appropriateness of the dosage form.

Patients may not comply with therapy because they do not understand what it is for or what is required of them. Asking the Public Health Service screening questions in Chapter 3 will give pharmacists ample evidence if this is the source of noncompliance.

Finally, some patients are deliberately noncompliant. They may feel that the medication is not working or is causing more problems than it treats, they may have a different goal for therapy than the pharmacist or physician does, or they may simply not want to take the drug. Having to take a drug reminds patients that there is something wrong with them, and some may find that hard to acknowledge.

Changing drugs on the basis of cost alone is not always wise.

BOX 4-2

Compliance Is a Patient's Decision

Education and reassurance may not always be enough to motivate patients to comply with drug therapy. Pharmacists must work with patients to help them see the benefits of therapy and must be considerate of their fears and concerns. Sometimes, the underlying issue can be identified and addressed, such as the medication's cost or the patient's difficulty swallowing it. Many times, however, it becomes a patient's personal decision to comply.

Simple education and reassurance may not always be enough to motivate such patients to comply with therapy. The pharmacist needs to work with them to help them see the benefits of therapy and must also be considerate of their fears and concerns. Sometimes, the underlying issue can be identified and readily addressed, but ultimately it becomes a patient's personal decision to comply. Despite the pharmacist's good faith effort to educate the patient and the patient's apparent understanding, the patient may still refuse drug therapy. Then the problem is not manageable until the patient accepts it as a problem.

Adverse Effects and Drug Interactions

Assessment of adverse effects and drug interactions is discussed last. Most problems of this nature will be revealed during the evaluation as the pharmacist examines the patient's response to drug therapy. Adverse effects related to drugs not considered safe for the patient should be found when determining if the patient is on the right drug. Similarly, adverse effects caused by rapid changes in dose or improper drug administration should be found when the dose and dosage form are evaluated.

BOX 4-3

Disagreements on What to Call a Problem

Although pharmacists and physicians will generally agree on the existence of a problem, they will frequently disagree on what to call it. For example, if a patient with a history of bleeding ulcers suffers gastric pain after taking prednisone for asthma, is the problem "unsafe drug for patient," "adverse effect," "inappropriate dosage form," or something else?

Pharmacists are encouraged to identify all the possible ways they could categorize potential problems and work through them for errors in logic, interpretation of patient data, or literature. After this process, several equally valid choices may remain. In such cases, the nature of the problem is frequently dictated by the nature of the care plan. Essentially, the exact cause of the problem is defined retrospectively.

In the previous example, if taking the prednisone with an antacid is thought to be a valid recommendation, then the problem could be fairly characterized as an adverse effect or a need for additional therapy. If another pharmacist suggests that the prednisone could be safely changed to a steroid inhaler, then identifying the problem as an incorrect dosage form may be more reasonable.

Although different pharmacists may never come to consensus on the strict definition of a problem, they should become comfortable in defending their conclusions based on interpretation of patient-specific and literature-based data. Pharmacists should not be overly concerned about coming to a consensus; rather, they should be sure that they have identified all the patient's problems.

The one type of adverse effect that must be identified separately is related to drug allergy. As pharmacists evaluate the patient, they must consider if any of the patient's conditions could be explained by an allergic reaction to a medication.

As we will see in Chapter 5, once drug therapy problems are identified, they must be prioritized. Not all the problems identified will be ones the pharmacist chooses to correct. But initially pharmacists should identify all possible problems and then decide which ones actually merit further attention. Once you become expert at identifying drug therapy problems, you will be able to edit the list in your mind.

Self Assessment Questions

These questions refer to the patient case in Table 4-1.

4.1 Compare Mrs. Rifkin's medication list to the list of medical conditions listed in her chart and any other diseases, signs, symptoms, or complaints she mentioned during the patient interview. What do you conclude?

4.2 Evaluate if Mrs. Rifkin may have any untreated indications by determining what is being done to treat each of her diseases, conditions, symptoms or complaints. What do you conclude?

4.3 Determine if each of Mrs. Rifkin's medications has an appropriate indication. What do you conclude?

4.4 What are your final conclusions? Does Mrs. Rifkin have any drug therapy problems related to appropriate indication or no untreated indications?

4.5 Evaluate the dose of each of Mrs. Rifkin's medications. Is there any evidence to suggest she has any actual or potential drug therapy problems related to the dose or dosage schedule of her medications? What do you conclude?

4.6 Evaluate the duration of therapy for each of Mrs. Rifkin's medications. What do you conclude?

4.7 Evaluate the dosage form for each of Mrs. Rifkin's medications. What do you conclude?

4.8 Is each of Mrs. Rifkin's medications the right/best one for each of her conditions? Are there any contraindications? Are any of her conditions refractory to drug therapy? Is more effective therapy available?

4.9 Does Mrs. Rifkin have any compliance-related drug therapy problems?

4.10 Does Mrs. Rifkin have any drug therapy problems related to adverse effects or drug interactions?

4.11 List all of the potential and actual drug therapy problems and their causes you found in Mrs. Rifkin.

Patient Care Plan Development
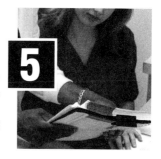

John P. Rovers

A care plan is a course of action for helping a patient achieve a particular health-related goal. In a way care plans are the "product" that the pharmaceutical care practitioner delivers; that is, a concrete process for optimizing a patient's health and well-being.

There are three basic components to a care plan: a goal for therapy, a plan to achieve the goal, and a plan to monitor the patient. These are the final three steps shown in the Pharmaceutical Care Cycle (see Figure 2-1).

To create a care plan, the pharmacist works with the patient (and often with other health care providers) to identify, evaluate, and choose methods for ensuring that drug therapy is effective and health-related problems are minimized. After completing a systematic evaluation of the patient, the pharmacist actively considers the patient's needs and determines desirable outcomes that both the pharmacist and patient agree on. The activities necessary to achieve these outcomes are then synthesized into a care plan, which the pharmacist documents in the patient's pharmacy record. When the situation warrants, the pharmacist reviews the plan and desirable outcomes with the patient's other health care providers.

In this chapter, the following concepts are reviewed:

- Prioritizing drug therapy problems.

- Setting therapeutic goals.

- Defining patient-focused interventions.

- Defining drug-focused interventions.

- Implementing care plans.

- Monitoring patients' treatment and follow-up.

BOX 5-1

A New Way of Practicing

Developing a care plan is absolutely vital to pharmacists providing pharmaceutical care. Although pharmacists have always gathered at least some patient information and found occasional drug therapy problems, they did not routinely develop a means by which to resolve problems. Instead, they would simply inform the physician of the problem and let him decide what should be done. In contrast, pharmaceutical care requires pharmacists to accept responsibility for a patient's drug-related outcomes.

Patients with multiple diseases or conditions may have care plans with various components. To make good decisions, the patient should be educated about the pros and cons of drug therapy options, such as cost, side effects, and monitoring-related factors. Of course, pharmacists should feel free to offer their professional judgment about the options that are the most beneficial. Essential elements of the plan, including the patient's responsibilities in carrying it out, must be carefully and completely explained to increase the likelihood of compliance. Ultimately, the patient must agree with the care plan the pharmacist develops. If patients object to their care plans they are less likely to adhere and may have a poor outcome.

Prioritizing Problems

After the pharmacist has identified all the patient's drug therapy problems, it is time to prioritize them according to their importance in the care process. As discussed in the case in Chapter 4 (see Self Assessment 4.11), an all inclusive list of a patient's drug therapy problems will generally include ones that overlap or turn out not to be problems at all. An initial screen of the patient's drug therapy problem list should be done to determine if there are duplications or areas that will be unlikely to require the pharmacist's attention. Then the pharmacist can create a prioritized list of problems that consist of those she genuinely needs to work on.

The following criteria should be taken into consideration when setting priorities:

• Acuity of problems.

• Seriousness of problems.

• Patient's perceptions of seriousness and urgency of problems.

• Potential to correct problems.

• Appropriateness of the pharmacist's addressing these problems.

Defining these criteria may help pharmacists use them properly. An acute problem is one that has a sudden onset, worsens quickly, and runs a brief course. It may or may not be life threatening, but time is of the essence and the pharmacist must solve this problem quickly. A serious problem is one that is nontrivial. It may even be life threatening. However, time is usually available to solve the problem; it does not necessarily need to be addressed immediately.

Using these definitions, a pharmacist can prioritize the patient's problems. To determine if any given problem is acute, serious, or both, she can ask herself, "Do I have time to solve this problem or will bad things happen if I wait?" If she doesn't have much time, then the problem is acute. Then she can ask, "Will bad things happen if I never solve this problem?" If so, the problem is serious.

Surprisingly, "actual" and "potential" are not criteria explicitly used to prioritize drug therapy problems. This is because potential problems, although they can be serious (e.g., drug interactions with warfarin) are usually not acute. Potential drug therapy problems, by definition, have not yet occurred, which means the pharmacist will have some time to prevent them. Actual drug therapy problems are more likely to be acute, thereby necessitating the pharmacist's immediate action to resolve them. Considerations of acuity and seriousness are more useful in problem prioritization than the actual or potential nature of the problem.

A problem that is both acute and serious is categorized as Priority I and should be addressed first. There is no time to lose. A problem that is acute but not serious is a Priority II problem. Although the problem may not be life threatening, time is not on your side. Finally, problems that are serious but not acute are designated Priority III. The problem is unlikely to be life threatening right at this very minute. Priority III problems can usually wait until you have solved the Priority I and II problems. Problems that are neither serious nor acute are also designated as Priority III.

The patient's perceptions of the seriousness and acuity of the problems are factored in when developing care plans for a patient with several Priority II or III problems. If the patient has

BOX 5-2

Solve Multiple Problems One at a Time

When patients have multiple drug therapy problems, pharmacists sometimes take on too much and try to solve them all at once. This is almost never the best approach. In many cases, a patient will have suffered from the problems for a considerable period of time. Except when problems are both acute and serious, pharmacists usually have time to address them one by one.

When pharmacists try to do too much at once, it is generally not clear which interventions resulted in which outcomes. Thus it can be hard to assess each outcome and determine if another intervention is needed. Usually pharmacists should address one or two problems at a time and come back to the remaining problems later.

multiple lower priority problems, they can usually be solved according to the patient's preference.

When these criteria are used properly, it becomes apparent that the most serious problem does not necessarily have to be addressed first. Consider a patient with prostate cancer whose disease has not fully responded to chemotherapy and has metastasized to the bones. An oral narcotic is controlling his bone pain well, but has led to severe constipation. Since his bone pain is currently well controlled, the pain does not represent a drug therapy problem at present. The patient's two drug therapy problems are:

• He needs additional therapy for his cancer.

• He suffers from the adverse effect of constipation caused by a narcotic.

A key question to consider is whether a problem is correctable by a pharmacist using the tools she has available.

The patient's most serious problem is the first one, since it has the most potential for a poor outcome—in this case, death. His most acute problem, however, is constipation. Because the clinical course of his cancer is likely to be much slower than the progression of complaints secondary to constipation, his bowel problems may be addressed before the cancer-related problems. The cancer is serious, but the constipation is more acute. In the short term it is likely to have a greater negative impact on this patient's quality of life than his life-threatening cancer. So in this case, the first problem of needing additional therapy is serious but not acute (Priority III) and the second problem is acute, but not serious (Priority II). This patient does not have any Priority I (both serious and acute) problems.

The last two criteria on the priority-setting list above are also important in this case. Problems related to cancer or pain management may be beyond a particular pharmacist's level of competence and expertise. Using the average pharmacist's expertise at creating care plans for bone pain, the problem has a low potential to be solved. So it would be best for the pharmacist to focus on the patient's constipation since she may be the most appropriate health professional to resolve it.

A key question to consider is whether a problem is correctable by a pharmacist using the tools she has available. If the patient in the bone pain example above should require radiation treatment, his pharmacist would not be able to correct the problem with drug therapy (the problem is not correctable from a pharmacist's perspective). The problem would be a low-priority one, but this does not necessarily mean it is insignificant.

In addition, a low-priority problem for the pharmacist may be a high-priority problem for the patient or physician. If it is, the pharmacist cannot ignore the problem but must refer the patient to the provider best suited to solve it. All providers need to work together with the common goal of resolving all the patient's drug therapy and medical problems.

Most ambulatory patients will have only one drug therapy problem. In some patients, however, the pharmacist will find multiple problems and need to prioritize them. This is especially true in hospitalized patients.

Setting Therapeutic Goals

After screening and prioritizing the patient's drug therapy problems, the next step in developing a care plan is determining the outcome the pharmacist hopes to achieve for each problem. In other words, the pharmacist should establish therapeutic goals and make sure they are acceptable to the patient. If the patient and pharmacist do not have similar goals, the patient is unlikely to comply with the care plan.

Goals are not often explicit. Ideally the pharmacist will write them down in the patient's pharmaceutical care record, but in most cases they are simply a concept that the pharmacist keeps in mind while developing a care plan. If that is the case, then why have them?

Goals are important for two reasons. First, without having at least a mental concept of what his goal is, a pharmacist will have difficulty making the best choices to achieve it. Second, being able to articulate a goal will help ensure that a pharmacist stays within her scope of practice. Well structured goals will always be worded in such a way as to focus on drugs and drug therapy problems.

Sometimes the goals a patient has in mind are unrealistic, so the pharmacist must provide significant education to help the patient understand what may be accomplished. Other times, the patient's goals are not unreasonable, but simply different from those of the pharmacist or physician.

For example, a patient prescribed a cholesterol-lowering agent to be taken twice daily had the goal of taking only one tablet per day. On this therapy, he reduced his cholesterol from 430 mg/dL to 260 mg/dL. From the patient's perspective, this drop in cholesterol was sufficient to lower his cholesterol (plus it met his desire to take only one pill daily). Although the pharmacist tried to impress upon the patient that a further decrease in serum cholesterol was highly desirable, the patient remained unconvinced. Since his goals were being met, he had little interest in the goals of the pharmacist or physician.

The pharmacist must also consider the physician's goals for therapy. Sometimes these may not be readily apparent or they may not be explicit. In such cases, the pharmacist will need to inform the physician of the pharmaceutical goals for therapy to ensure that the pharmacist and physician are not working at cross-purposes.

Even when the patient, pharmacist, and physician have mutual goals, they may phrase them differently so that they appear to be dissimilar. Pharmacists should look carefully for areas of common interest. For example, a patient with poorly controlled diabetes had significant nocturia. The physician's goal was to decrease the patient's bedtime serum glucose level, and the pharmacist wanted to improve the patient's quality of life. The patient simply claimed he wanted "to stop peeing at night." Although these goals all sound very different, they were readily reconciled so that each party achieved his goal by using a mutually agreeable care plan.

Ill-Defined Goals

The first few times a pharmacist develops patient-specific goals, they tend to be vague. Pharmacists must ensure that their goals are achievable, measurable, and consistent with their professional responsibilities. For example, after interviewing and evaluating a patient with poorly controlled hypertension, secondary to poor

BOX 5-3

Pharmaceutical Care Goals May Differ from "Traditional" Goals

Many pharmacists first learn about "goals" in therapeutics class, and some, especially clinically oriented practitioners, are accustomed to working with physicians to establish goals for therapy. Although the goals taught in therapeutics courses or set by clinical pharmacists often complement the goals of pharmaceutical care practitioners, they tend to be more narrowly focused and are usually related to an objective parameter, such as a laboratory assessment.

Examples would be establishing a target hemoglobin A1c level for a patient with diabetes or setting a goal international normalized ratio for a patient on anticoagulant therapy. Although these are rational, defensible goals for therapy, most pharmacists do not participate in drug-use decision making at a level that involves them in setting such goals. Goals in pharmaceutical care are generally broader, which allows them to be set independent of the practice site.

medication compliance, a less experienced pharmacist may devise goals like "control patient's blood pressure" or "improve compliance." Although these seem reasonable, on further inspection it is apparent that there is no way to tell when such a goal has been accomplished. For instance, what does "improve" mean? Suppose the patient improves his compliance from taking 50% of doses correctly to 60%. Does this change mean the goal has been met?

Since the pharmacist has not explicitly defined her goals for the patient, there is no way to determine if they have been achieved. Blood pressures and compliance can be objectively evaluated and are measurable, but the target measures have not been stated.

An experienced pharmaceutical care practitioner would probably state the goals this way:

- "The patient demonstrates an understanding of the need for compliance with his drug therapy and refills 80% of his prescriptions within 5 days of the appropriate refill date."

- "The patient will experience slowed progression of hypertension complications by taking enough of his medication to maintain BP < 140/90."

Since the pharmacist should readily be able to educate the patient about the risks of uncontrolled hypertension and the importance of compliance, such goals are achievable. They are measurable, since the refill target date is explicitly stated and easily evaluated, and blood pressure is easily monitored. They are also consistent with the responsibilities of the pharmaceutical care provider.

TABLE 5-1

Defining Goals

Pharmacists must ensure that their goals are:

- Achievable.

- Measurable.

- Consistent with their professional responsibilities.

The example above also demonstrates how to develop a goal for an outcome that is not really measurable. If a patient has gastric upset from a nonsteroidal anti-inflammatory agent, there is no truly objective method to measure his level of pain relief. Therefore the measurement becomes either the patient's voiced complaints or his level of understanding. For the patient with hypertension, the phrase "the patient demonstrates" is as good a measure as can be defined. For the patient with gastric pain, a statement that "the patient no longer complains of stomach pain" defines the measurement. If a goal cannot be readily measured, it should focus on the patient's greater understanding of the situation or subjective decrease in symptoms.

Confusing Goals with Methods

As pharmacists learn to set goals for therapy, they sometimes confuse the goal with its method of implementation by defining the care plan as the goal. For example, suppose a pharmacist evaluating a patient learns that red wine is a consistent trigger for her migraine headaches. The goal of therapy is not to educate the patient and convince her to stop drinking red wine. That is the plan. The goal is that the patient no longer complains of unacceptable numbers of migraine headaches.

One quick way to determine if you have created a goal or a care plan is to write it down. Then, look at the main verb in the sentence and see to whom it applies. In the first example above, the "goal" was to educate the patient. Since the pharmacist will be providing the education, the verb "educate" applies to the pharmacist. In the second example, the verb "complain" applies to the patient.

In other words, if the verb in your goal statement applies to the pharmacist, it's almost certainly a plan, not a goal. If the verb applies to the patient, then you have properly documented a goal. Although the distinction between goal and plan may seem obvious, in practice pharmacists frequently confuse the two.

Compound Goals

Some pharmacists create more complex goals than the example shown above. These can be called compound goals. In a compound goal, the pharmacist recognizes that her care plan may result in a therapeutic (i.e., beneficial) outcome but may also result in an adverse outcome. Compound goals are written to make it explicit that a therapeutic outcome is desired, without an adverse outcome developing at the same time.

For example, suppose that the patient above with migraine headaches needed to be treated with sumatriptan. A possible compound goal in this case would be, "The patient will express adequate relief from her migraine headaches without developing adverse effects from sumatriptan such as dizziness or chest pain."

Although compound goals may not always be necessary, they show that the pharmacist has used a rigorous thought process in creating a goal for the patient.

Overview of Care Planning

Once pharmacists have developed a care plan, they have completed the third step in the Pharmaceutical Care Cycle. While creating the plan, the pharmacist integrates everything she knows about patients, their pathophysiology, the social or economic factors that relate to their health, the health care system, and drugs—including pharmacology, therapeutics, chemistry, and dosage forms. Care plan development requires that pharmacists consider all these elements and use them to identify the best way to resolve the patient's drug therapy problems.

Initially, pharmacists should consider all possible interventions to make the best choice. They should ask themselves, "Given everything I know about this patient, the health care system, and drug therapy, what are all the possible things I could do?" Then they should ask, "Out of all these options, what is the best thing for me to do?"

TABLE 5-2

List All Options before Choosing the Best

When developing care plans, pharmacists should not edit their options immediately. They can write down several things that they could do to solve the problem. This way, they are more likely to choose the best option, not just the most apparent one. For example, in a patient who suffers from stomach pain after taking a nonsteroidal anti-inflammatory drug the pharmacist could:

• Recommend he take it with food.

• Suggest the patient change to a COX-2 inhibitor such as celecoxib.

• Suggest that misoprostol be added to the regimen.

• Stop drug therapy altogether and monitor for what happens next.

Depending on patient-specific circumstances, any one of these four choices may be appropriate. Data from the patient history will point the pharmacist to the best choice.

When considering options, pharmacists should evaluate possible alternatives and work with patients and often with other health care providers to choose the best course. There are usually at least two options for every drug therapy problem.

If drug therapy is to be modified, the pharmacist should investigate therapeutic alternatives in order to balance efficacy, safety, and cost. Taking the time to know the patient and develop a professional relationship will make weighing these factors easier. Cost or complexity of therapy may affect some patients' compliance, as may the psychosocial aspects of a disease or specific patient preferences.

Poor Care Plans

When pharmacists devise a poor care plan, it is typically because they have not taken the time to reflect on everything they know and examine their options. The first reasonable method for resolving the patient's drug therapy problem becomes the care plan. The most obvious intervention may not always be the best one.

The most obvious intervention may not always be the best one.

For example, in a patient with significant esophageal strictures who has extreme difficulty swallowing most solid dosage forms, the most obvious plan would be switching to a liquid dosage form. But because liquid dosage forms are often more expensive than equipotent doses of a tablet or capsule, this "obvious" care plan may not be the best one for a patient on a limited income and without prescription insurance. Another "obvious" care plan, such as having the patient crush the tablet and take it in jelly, would be equally irrational when dealing with a sustained release product that must not be crushed.

A care plan must start by ensuring that the patient needs the drug. If he does not, then the issue of dosage form is irrelevant. Pharmacists developing care plans must be sure they use all the information available to avoid settling for easy answers that may not be best for the patient.

TABLE 5-3

Developing Care Plans: Questions to Ask Yourself

- Given everything I know about this patient, the health care system, and drug therapy, what are all the possible things I could do?

- Out of all these options, what is the best thing for me to do?

Additional Research

Sometimes additional research may be necessary to come to a decision about drug therapy options. Areas the pharmacist may need to research include:

• The patient's disease.

• Consequences to the patient of a particular drug therapy program.

• Usual drug and nondrug therapies.

• Dosages, adverse effects, and interactions of usual therapies.

After researching, the pharmacist should consider how the patient's unique combination of characteristics fits into the "big picture" of the disease states and conditions. Consider patients with cystitis. Although the underlying pathophysiology, consequences of infection, and general antibiotic choices will be similar in most cases, those who are pregnant, on theophylline, are catheterized, have drug allergies, or have had multiple infections have special considerations that make their management unique. The choice of drug, dosage interval, or duration of therapy may differ for different patients even if they suffer from the same condition. If the pharmacist is not aware of how patients' specific conditions may affect their care plans, it is necessary to research the possible options and choose the best one.

Patient-Focused Interventions

As pharmacists begin to gain expertise at developing care plans, they soon see that two basic types of interventions may be made: patient-focused or drug-focused.

Patient-focused interventions include assisting the patient with compliance problems, providing patient education, monitoring the patient, and implementing nondrug therapy such as a weight control program. Patient-focused interventions typically do not require the physician's permission to implement. Nevertheless, most pharmacists elect to keep physicians informed about patient-focused interventions and the drug therapy problems being targeted.

Some patient-focused interventions may be quite in-depth and formalized. This may be especially true for pharmacists who offer disease management programs for asthma, weight loss, or other conditions. A well-designed disease management program will include specific educational or patient-monitoring interventions that the pharmacist will perform in a consistent, systematic fashion. In an asthma program, for example, the pharmacist may teach the patient about dust control, pets, asthma triggers, smoking cessation, peak flow monitoring, or inhaler technique— interventions that are entirely educational and not related to a drug. These interventions would be presented as well-designed plans with defined outcomes, not casual discussions between pharmacist and patient.

Educational interventions need not always be so complex. For example, most pharmacists will not establish a formal compliance clinic. Instead, they will provide general education on the patient's drugs and diseases, discuss the need for compliance, and perhaps furnish compliance aids such as pill boxes or dosing calendars.

Patient-focused interventions may also involve referring a patient for medical care. Although pharmacists have performed this service for years, in a pharmaceutical care practice they are able to provide additional information to let the physician know how they evaluated the problem; what, if anything, has been done about it so far; and what recommendations the pharmacist has.

When a pharmacist intends to make a drug-related intervention, it is important to be specific.

Drug-Focused Interventions

Drug-focused interventions require some type of change in a patient's drug therapy. Potential changes are adding, discontinuing, or changing a drug, or changing a dose, dosage interval, or dosage form. Unless the drug-focused intervention involves a nonprescription medication, most will require the physician's cooperation to implement.

When a pharmacist intends to make a drug-related intervention, it is important to be specific. Recommendations that are too vague are not useful. For example, suggesting to a physician that a patient with early diabetes-related renal impairment be started on an angiotensin-converting enzyme (ACE) inhibitor is not very helpful because it makes the physician responsible for choosing the drug, dose, dosage form, and duration of therapy. Pharmacists must make their suggestions as explicit as possible, even if it requires considerable time to research a disease and its treatment. A good drug-focused recommendation will focus on one drug, not an entire therapeutic category.

Plus making a nonspecific suggestion raises the possibility that the physician could choose a therapy which results in a new drug-related problem. For example, if the pharmacist simply suggested that the physician start the patient with early renal impairment on captopril, the physician might choose too low a dose.

Making multiple, detailed suggestions is equally unhelpful to the physician and the patient. (In other words, having too many choices is as bad as having too few.) For the patient needing an ACE inhibitor, for example, clinical pharmacists might suggest half a dozen alternative drugs, dosages, and dosage schedules. Physicians are then left to choose which alternative is the best without having the information or resources they need to make that choice. When providing multiple suggestions, pharmacists may wish to prioritize their recommendations but have a next-best alternative in mind.

When considering drug-related interventions, pharmacists should be aware of making too many changes at once. Since drugs have such powerful and complex effects, the therapeutic response for one condition may result in an adverse effect on another condition. Ideally, pharmacists work with physicians to observe the response to one change in drug therapy before embarking on a second change. Some patients will be sufficiently ill that multiple drug-related interventions are indicated, but in most patients, one change at a time is usually the better plan.

"Do Nothing" Interventions

One final form of intervention is not really drug- or patient-focused. Historically pharmacists did not identify and resolve drug therapy problems in a consistent manner, so the "do nothing" option was a default action when they were not aware that something had to be done. In a pharmaceutical care practice, however, "do nothing" is a considered, deliberate decision resulting from the pharmacist's determination that no action is better than doing anything else. It is a form of patient monitoring similar to the "watchful waiting" described in Chapter 4. Although the "do nothing" option is rarely the correct choice for a patient, it should be considered and deliberately ruled out before proceeding to other interventions.

Final Steps

One of the last steps in developing a care plan is formulating a strategy for measuring whether the proposed outcomes have been achieved. This strategy should provide both objective and subjective information. Finally, the pharmacist should review the plan with the patient, indicating specifically what outcomes the patient should expect from drug therapy. It is very important for the pharmacist to speak at the appropriate level for the patient and make sure the patient understands how to incorporate the drug therapy into his or her everyday life. To ensure patient understanding, it is helpful to ask the patient to explain the process back to the pharmacist.

Implementing Care Plans

When providing pharmaceutical care, it is essential to ensure that the patient has the means to comply with the pharmacist's care plan. In other words, the pharmacist must verify that the patient has the drugs, supplies, and information necessary to carry out the plan. If verification does not take place and the care plan is not properly implemented, the desired goals for therapy will not be achieved.

It should not be assumed that once the pharmacist has told the patient what to do, the patient will do it. If patients are left to gather supplies, contact the physician, and then go home to decide how to proceed, they may not be able to follow the pharmacist's care plan. Implementing a care plan is a cooperative effort. The pharmacist must coordinate between the patient and physician to be certain that all parties understand what is required of them and that they know when various aspects of patient care and monitoring will occur.

Patient-Focused Care Plans

Implementing a patient-focused care plan is not particularly complicated, especially if the pharmacist has established a therapeutic relationship with a patient who has consented to follow the plan. It only remains for the pharmacist to:

• Verify the patient's understanding of the plan.

• See that the patient has the necessary drugs and supplies.

• Make sure that the patient understands the need for follow-up.

• Make sure the patient will participate in monitoring.

On occasion, pharmacists may perform these activities with patients' family members or another caregiver if, for example, the patient is a child or is elderly and incapacitated. Since the physician is not typically involved to any great extent with a patient-focused care plan, the pharmacist usually needs only to inform the physician of what was done, not gain permission to proceed.

Ensure Understanding

When making sure that patients have a good understanding of their drug therapy, the pharmacist must verify that they know how to take their medications and then correct any misperceptions. Thinking back to the three Public Health Service questions in Chapter 3 is helpful (see page 56). During the patient interview, patients should have been able to explain to the pharmacist how much they understand about what the medications are for, exactly how to take them, and what to expect. If, during the patient interview, the pharmacist learns that a patient does not understand these basics, then correcting knowledge deficits becomes an initial step in implementing the care plan.

Tailoring explanations to the patient's level of comprehension is critical. In some cases, pharmacists may need to employ teaching aids, such as visual devices, graphics, or brochures, to supplement instruction. The best teaching technique is modeling; if possible, have the patient demonstrate the correct administration of the drug. To test patient understanding, the pharmacist should have the pa-

BOX 5-4

Pharmacists' Fears in Care Planning

Pharmacists often hesitate to devise and implement care plans until they feel they are pharmaceutical care experts. This may be because they may lack confidence in their therapeutic knowledge base or patient management skills. Pharmacists who do not yet feel comfortable with pharmaceutical care may decide that action is not indicated and that they will "monitor" the patient until the problem appears serious enough to require further intervention. This is a misuse of the term "monitoring." The pharmacist is responding to a fear that by doing something he could actually make things worse.

Although such fears are not unreasonable, most pharmacists never consider that not acting also carries a potential for risk. The literature suggests that a substantial number of hospital admissions are because of drugs, and that drug therapy problems cost the U.S. health care system billions of dollars a year. According to a report published by the Institute of Medicine in 2000,[1] as many as 98,000 Americans die each year as a result of medical mistakes. That's a loss of life equivalent to a full Boeing 747 crashing every other day for an entire year. A follow up report from the Institute of Medicine published in 2006 revealed that at least 1.5 million preventable adverse drug reactions occur annually in the U.S.[2] Pharmacists are well positioned to assist with these problems, but to do so, they must act.

Pharmacists must remember that although pharmaceutical care draws on knowledge of drugs and diseases, the two are not synonymous. Pharmacists trained in pharmaceutical care have repeatedly demonstrated the ability to find and resolve drug therapy problems irrespective of their knowledge base, age, practice setting, or pharmacy degree. The more pharmacists know about drugs and diseases, the more problems they will find, and the more varied their solutions will be. All pharmacists have the basic tools to find and resolve at least some drug therapy problems and do good things for patients.

Fearful pharmacists might consider the maxim, "Do not let the perfect be the enemy of the good." If pharmacists wait until we are entirely comfortable with all aspects of care planning before intervening in patient care, the serious drug-related problems facing the health care system will not be resolved. If there are 98,000 fatalities and 1.5 million adverse effects every year, is one pharmacist likely to make things worse?

BOX 5-5

To ensure understanding, patients should be asked to repeat instructions back to the pharmacist. A pharmacist might request, "To be sure I didn't leave out anything important, would you mind telling me [or showing me] how you will use your medication?"

tient explain the information back and show the pharmacist how to administer the drug. Some patients may become irritated at being asked to repeat explanations, interpreting this request as a suggestion that the pharmacist thinks they did not understand the teaching. Pharmacists may wish to preface their request by stating that this is done to ensure that the pharmacist did not leave anything out.

Educating patients about their diseases may be handled in a similar way. Such education is especially important for patients with compliance problems related to misunderstandings about their medical condition. Typically, it is while educating patients about their diseases that care plans related to lifestyle modifications are put into effect.

Lifestyle-Related Plans

Lifestyle-related care plans are common since virtually everyone agrees on the wisdom of losing weight, stopping smoking, eating right, and getting more sleep and exercise. However, these are among the most difficult interventions for pharmacists to implement and for patients to comply with. Patient-focused interventions that involve lifestyle changes require ongoing patient contact and reassurance.

Formal disease management programs are attractive when lifestyle changes are part of the plan because they give both the pharmacist and patient a series of steps to follow. Informally encouraging patients to stop smoking or lose weight is rarely successful; most people already know they should make these changes. As with drug therapy education, the pharmacist should use whatever tools are helpful and then be sure that the patient demonstrates understanding.

Monitoring Mechanisms

Working with patients to develop and implement monitoring mechanisms helps ensure that they can and will comply with the necessary drug therapy or disease monitoring. If objective drug therapy monitoring tools such as laboratory testing, blood pressure monitoring, peak flow meters, or home glucose monitors will be employed, the pharmacist should see that arrangements for this monitoring have been made and are understood by the patient. This may include obtaining devices, explaining their use, and keeping records that the pharmacist or physician can evaluate with the patient during follow-up sessions. Again, demonstrating the equipment and having the patient explain back and show correct usage is an excellent way to determine if the patient will be able to carry out the monitoring plan.

Complex Cases

For patients with more complicated diseases and therapies, pharmacists may have to implement a patient-focused care plan that includes several steps at the same time. For example, diabetic patients who require insulin and home blood glucose testing should be educated about:

• The effects of insulin on their disease state.

• Timing and amount of insulin injected.

• Correct injection technique.

• Correct storage of insulin.

• Overall expected results.

• Side effects of insulin.

• How to counteract a hypoglycemic reaction.

• Precautions necessary for diabetics on insulin.

The pharmacist should also make sure that patients possess the appropriate home blood glucose testing equipment and supplies and know how to use them, have the necessary medications and insulin syringes, and understand—and are willing and able to fulfill—their therapy plans.

Final Check

The last step is a final check to ensure that all the patient's follow-up activities are coordinated. The pharmacist must verify that:

• Patients have set up any necessary follow-up appointments with their physicians.

BOX 5-6

Verifying Drugs, Supplies

Verifying that the patient has, or can obtain, all the necessary drugs, devices, and supplies necessary to follow the care plan is essential. This activity is especially important when patients will use a different source for these goods than the pharmacist who is providing pharmaceutical care. The pharmacist should also consider the patient's financial and insurance status to be certain they do not represent barriers to following a care plan.

- Patients know where and when to report for further laboratory monitoring.

- A date, time, and mechanism have been established for follow-up with the pharmacist.

Drug-Focused Care Plans

With the exception of care plans related to nonprescription medications, drug-focused care plans usually require the physician's cooperation. Consequently, they are more complex

---

BOX 5-7

Propose Solutions to Develop Professional Relationships with Physicians

For pharmacists to work cooperatively with physicians, a mutually respectful professional relationship is necessary. Unfortunately, some pharmacist–physician relationships lack this quality. This may be because the most common contact physicians have with pharmacists, outside of prescription refill requests, is when pharmacists call to inform them of patient allergies, previous adverse effects, conflicts with third-party formularies, or patients who cannot afford a drug. In each case, the pharmacist is informing the physician of a problem.

The potential unspoken message is that the physician erred in prescribing, or else this problem would not have happened. Pharmacists do not intend to convey this message but it is largely unavoidable. If every phone call pharmacists received from physicians pointed out dispensing problems, pharmacists would not want to talk to physicians very much, either.

When pharmacists call to point out a problem, they rarely describe it succinctly, outline why it is important to both the patient and the physician, and then recommend a resolution that is based on patient-specific knowledge. Instead, pharmacists typically let physicians know there is a problem and then fall silent. To the unspoken message, "You made a mistake," the pharmacist adds, "And what do you propose to do about it?"

Although pharmaceutical care practice still requires that pharmacists inform physicians of drug therapy problems, smart practitioners try to change the dynamics of the relationship.

- They meet with local physicians to inform them of changes they are making in their practices to better assist their mutual patients.

- They explain how pharmacists can help physicians by taking over some of the time-consuming educational activities that busy physicians may not have time for.

- They consistently demonstrate that they are making these changes to help patients.

Even practitioners who are not able to actively market themselves to the local medical community can take a vital step to change the pharmacist–physician relationship: Whenever they contact a physician to discuss a drug therapy problem, they propose a solution. Once physicians understand that pharmacists are interested in and capable of solving problems, rather than just pointing them out, a relationship between professional colleagues is likely to ensue.

---

to implement. The first step is ensuring that the patient understands and has agreed to the drug-therapy changes that the pharmacist has proposed. Then the pharmacist can contact the physician to propose the changes. These suggestions must be as specific as possible. Pharmacists should outline their recommendations to physicians in the following areas:

- Drug.

- Dose.

- Dosage form.

- Duration of therapy.

- Appropriate monitoring parameters.

- Who will perform the monitoring and when.

Patients Delivering Care Plans

There are several ways to contact the physician to implement a care plan. Often patients will insist that they see the physician themselves and discuss the pharmacist's care plan directly with the doctor. This scenario is most likely when there is no urgent or serious problem that needs immediate correction or when the patient has a scheduled physician appointment coming up soon. Pharmacists must be respectful of such patient preferences. Information from patient focus groups has shown that, although patients support the concept of pharmaceutical care and appreciate the pharmacist's actions, they clearly do not want the pharmacist to interfere with the physician–patient relationship.

When patients implement drug-focused care plans by communicating directly with their physicians, there is a risk that patients will deliver the pharmacist's message incorrectly, incompletely, or with the emphasis misplaced. Imagine the physician's response if the patient said, "The pharmacist told me to tell you to increase my dosage of metoprolol." When the patient insists on communicating with the physician herself, the best thing for the pharmacist to do is to write the physician a letter (and possibly include a SOAP note, see Chapter 6) and give it to the patient to take to the physician. This way, the message is more likely to be delivered as it was intended.

Patients may be curious as to what has been written about them and may wish to read any communications to the physician. By not writing anything they would be embarrassed to discuss with the patient in person and by placing correspondence in an unsealed envelope, pharmacists can assuage the patient's fears while still communicating professionally with the physician.

Discussing Plans by Phone

Most drug-focused care plans are implemented after the pharmacist has discussed the plan with the physician by telephone. This approach requires pharmacists to clearly organize the message they wish to send and how they want to send it. When contacting physicians by telephone, pharmacists must:

• Know what they want to say before making the call.

• Have at least one solution for every drug therapy problem discussed.

BOX 5-8

Communication Tip: Know What You Want to Say

Developing drug-focused care plans is sometimes easier than employing the communication skills necessary to implement them. Too often, pharmacists phone the physician's office before they have worked out everything they want to say. Even when they have established a defensible care plan, they may neglect to "sell" it to the physician appropriately.

For example, while interviewing a patient, a pharmacist learned that she had a painful condition that was being treated with an expensive drug. Although the drug worked well and was not causing any problems, the patient was on a fixed income and only took it when her symptoms were severe. Consequently, her disease was not being well controlled and she frequently had pain.

The pharmacist's care plan called for the expensive drug to be changed to a less expensive agent, and he contacted the physician to ask for permission to make the switch. The physician refused. The pharmacist was surprised; he had identified a serious problem and developed a good care plan. Why wouldn't the physician cooperate?

The physician's perspective was this: He had received a phone call from a pharmacist he did not know, about a patient he had not seen in several months, asking to change a medication that he was not aware was causing problems. This attempt to implement a care plan had no context.

Had the physician clearly understood that the patient's disease was poorly controlled because she could not afford her medicine, which therefore was not achieving the intended therapeutic effect, it would have made a big difference. Any reasonable physician recognizes that a poor outcome needs to be corrected. But the pharmacist did not outline the problem clearly, explain that he was using patient-specific knowledge, or emphasize that the problem was discovered by talking with the patient. If he had, the pharmacist's suggestion to change to a specific dosage of an alternative, and his offer to follow up with the patient to ensure that no further problems developed, would have been more warmly received.

A PRACTICAL GUIDE TO PHARMACEUTICAL CARE: A Clinical Skills Primer

- Consider ahead of time how the call may sound to a physician who is unaware that a problem exists.

Many pharmacists who try to telephone physicians express considerable frustration at not being able to navigate through the various layers of personnel in the medical office. They wonder if staff members actively try to prevent them from speaking with the physician (and may be surprised to learn that slowing down access to the physician is, indeed, part of their job). Because a physician's time is both scarce and expensive, there has to be a convincing reason to let the pharmacist through all the barriers. Too often the pharmacist does not provide one. Pharmacists who get through typically have developed a solid relationship with the physician and have demonstrated that it is worth the physician's time to accept their phone calls.

Some pharmacists get through by using drug-related jargon beyond the comprehension of receptionists and even some nurses. If office staff do not understand what the pharmacist is talking about but believe it to be serious, they may forward the call to the physician. (Pharmacists who use this approach must be absolutely certain of what they are talking about, so the technique is not recommended for beginners or for the fainthearted.)

Ultimately, the best way to get a message through is to be known by the physician and especially his office staff. Taking the time to meet with the doctor, nurses, receptionists, and other key personnel allows the pharmacist to become familiar with the office and discuss telephone procedures. If a pharmacist knows when a physician would prefer to be (or not to be) called and the physician knows the pharmacist will only contact him regarding important matters, their relationship can be a mutually respectful partnership.

Conveying Plans in Writing

A good method for sharing the care plan is to contact the physician in writing, either by fax or by mail. This method has many advantages:

- Writing down what they want to communicate to the physician allows pharmacists to think through the care plan thoroughly and to consider exactly what they want to tell the physician and the best way to say it.

- The physician can contemplate the pharmacist's suggestions at length without having to react immediately in response to a telephone call.

• The letter serves as a form of documentation that the pharmacist and physician can keep in the patient's chart as a record of their activities.

If the pharmacist is not an experienced writer, it may take several drafts to produce an acceptable letter. The pharmacist should be sure that the wording is clear and concise, yet thorough; that the problem is clearly stated; that a solution is proposed; and that nothing in the letter may inadvertently give offense. Words on a page do not communicate a person's emotions and tone as well as the voice does. A poor choice of written words may offend someone even when the same words delivered verbally do not cause problems.

Keep in mind that although written communication is efficient and avoids some potential pitfalls of telephone interventions, it is slower than other options and is not recommended for urgent problems that require immediate attention. If all of your interprofessional communications occur in writing, you may also find it harder to develop the level of trust in your abilities that the physicians you work with will require in order to be comfortable with your patient care practices.

Organizing Follow-up Monitoring

The final step in the Care Cycle is following up with the patient to monitor the outcome of the care plan. To ensure that specific goals are met, the pharmacist will need to regularly monitor the patient's progress according to the strategy outlined in the patient's drug therapy plan. At predetermined intervals the pharmacist will review subjective and objective monitoring parameters to determine if satisfactory progress is being made and if further drug therapy problems have developed. Patient monitoring is similar in some ways to the data gathering carried out during the initial pharmaceutical care visit, but is more focused.

If the desired outcomes are not being met, or if new problems have occurred, the pharmacist, physician, and patient may need to discuss possible changes in the drug therapy plan. Changes may be warranted to maintain or enhance the safety or effectiveness of drug therapy, or to minimize overall health care costs.

When to Follow Up

First, the pharmacist should determine exactly when to follow up on a patient's progress. Criteria to consider include:

- Expected time course before a therapeutic effect is seen.

- Expected time course before an adverse effect is seen.

- Time to onset of a possible drug interaction.

- Natural course of the disease.

- Length of time drug therapy will be required.

- Likelihood of additional drug therapy problems and their seriousness.

In establishing times to follow up with patients, the type of disease state and the patient's specific risk factors should be weighted heavily. For instance, patients taking medication for acute conditions may be contacted within a few hours or after several days, depending on the length and purpose of the drug therapy. However, patients taking medications for chronic conditions usually need to be contacted several times:

1. Five to 10 days after beginning therapy.

2. One month after initial follow-up.

3. Every 3 to 6 months during ongoing therapy.

Patients at a high risk of drug therapy problems may need more frequent follow-ups.

Patient Care Plan Development

To ensure that specific goals are met, the pharmacist will need to regularly monitor the patient's progress according to the strategy outlined in the patient's drug therapy plan.

Coordinating with the Patient

Next, the pharmacist needs to coordinate with the patient to establish a follow-up schedule and method. Because patients are not accustomed to having pharmacists monitor their clinical progress, it is important to inform them that a follow-up session is necessary. Patients who receive a phone call from the pharmacist without expecting one will tend to assume that there is a problem with their prescription. Or, if they are unaware that the pharmacist plans to call them and a third party answers, they may resent the loss of confidentiality. Patients have to know when the pharmacist will contact them and how.

Follow-up Approaches

The two basic approaches for patient follow-up are telephone calls and repeat visits to the pharmacy. When phone calls are to be used, the pharmacist must ensure that the patient's record includes the appropriate telephone number (home or workplace) and the best time to call. If the patient has particular concerns about confidentiality (as in the case of a teenage girl taking oral contraceptives) the record should also note whether it is acceptable to indicate to a third party that the pharmacist has called or whether it is permissible to leave a message.

If follow-up will be performed during a repeat visit to the pharmacy, it is best to use scheduled appointments. This ensures that the pharmacist knows the patient is coming in and has set aside time to perform the follow-up. The disadvantage to follow-up appointments is that patients often forget to keep them. It may be a good idea to call patients the day before an appointment to remind them; keep in mind, however, that telephone reminders also carry confidentiality risks.

Many pharmacists are initially concerned that they will need to do a follow-up evaluation each time the patient comes to the pharmacy for a prescription refill. However, most monitoring occurs at scheduled times. If a patient comes into the pharmacy between follow-up visits, the pharmacist should simply inquire briefly into the patient's progress by asking one or two open-ended questions, such as, "How has your drug therapy been working for you?" and "What new problems or concerns can I help you with?" If the medications seem to be working and the patient does not voice any new complaints, then the complete follow-up assessment can be performed as scheduled. If the patient indicates that there is a new drug therapy problem, the pharmacist can either address it immediately or move up the follow-up appointment.

After patients have been receiving pharmaceutical care for a while, they may be monitored by the pharmacist for several concurrent drug therapy problems. It is highly advisable to coordinate all follow-ups so that the pharmacist and patient do not need to schedule repeated sessions. Delaying some follow-ups for a few days or weeks will help prevent patients from losing interest in pharmaceutical care because of too many repeat visits close together.

Tracking Calls and Appointments

Pharmacists must have a mechanism for tracking which follow-ups need to be performed and when. The mechanism will depend on the pharmaceutical workload unique to each practice. At first, a simple wall or desk calendar may be used to write down the names and phone numbers of patients to contact. The first thing each morning, the pharmacist can check her schedule and prepare for the day's activities. The day before, the pharmacy technician should pull the files of all patients who will be seen the next day.

In busier practices, pharmacists are likely to use computer programs for documenting care, some of which have built-in calendar functions that set follow-up dates for patients and provide a written schedule of each day's activities. The technician can print out the appropriate information before a patient's visit, or the pharmacist can review the information on screen.

No matter how pharmacists follow up with patients, they should briefly review each patient's record before meeting with or telephoning the patient. Once they have more than a few pharmaceutical care patients in their practice, pharmacists often start to forget a patient's individual details. If patients get the impression that the pharmacist does not know the particulars of their case, it impairs the therapeutic relationship.

Information to Gather during Follow-up

Information the pharmacist needs to assess the effectiveness of therapy during a follow-up visit includes:

• Therapeutic efficacy of drug therapy.

• Safety of drug therapy.

• Drug interactions.

• Patient compliance.

• New problems of the patient.

• Unmet needs of the patient.

Answers to the questions to consider during monitoring (see Box 5-11) will show how well the care plan is working to achieve the therapeutic goals. They will also indicate if the drug therapy is causing any symptomatic adverse effects or drug interactions or if the patient has not complied with the care plan. As in the original data-gathering session described in Chapter 3, the pharmacist will collect both subjective and objective data and evaluate it. Once again, the pharmacist should start with open-ended questions and then narrow the scope with closed-ended questions. Unlike the pharmacist's initial interview with the patient, however, the questioning will focus more on drugs and diseases covered by the care plan.

If the pharmacist determines that the patient has not made clinical progress or that new drug therapy problems have arisen, she must work with the patient and physician to determine whether the original plan should be continued or modified. Some steps of the pharmaceutical care process may need to be repeated to help the patient work towards goals.

Continuing with the original care plan may be a good choice when there are compliance issues or when additional time may result in improvements. If the care plan is not working or if adverse effects or drug interactions have occurred, however, therapy may need to be modified.

If the initial interview showed that the patient's other diseases and drugs cause no problems, the follow-up visit need only confirm that no new problems have arisen with those diseases and drugs.

Only limited new data have to be collected during a follow-up session. The pharmacist should determine if patients have developed new medical conditions or have had changes in their drug therapy since the last visit. If they have, a focused interview should be performed to determine if the new diseases or changes in drug therapy have caused new drug therapy problems. Each time a new drug therapy problem is discovered, the Pharmaceutical Care Cycle begins again.

Progress toward Goals

Monitoring the patient's progress toward therapeutic goals involves comparing patient information with objective and subjective monitoring parameters. The patient's progress should be documented in the chart. When goals are being met, the pharmacist should give the patient positive reinforcement. This may take the form of cheerful encouragement or pointing out and congratulating a patient on marked improvement.

Self Assessment Questions

5.1 Below is the all-inclusive problem list previously created for Mrs. Rifkin, the patient in Chapter 4 (see Table 4-1). Screen this drug therapy problem list and develop a revised one that includes only those items that are likely to truly require the pharmacist's attention. Explain why you retained and deleted the problems you did.

Actual problems:

- "Adverse drug reaction" caused by undesirable effect caused by atenolol.

- "Dosage too low" caused by wrong dosage for calcium carbonate.

Potential problems:

- "Dosage too high" caused by wrong dosage for esomeprazole and acetaminophen, and also caused by duration inappropriate for esomeprazole.

- "Wrong drug" caused by more effective drug therapy available for esomeprazole.

- "Wrong drug" caused by contraindication present for EC ASA.

- "Needs additional drug therapy" caused by need for synergistic therapy with calcium and a biphosphonate.

Potential problems pending additional information:

- "No indication" caused by no medical indication for EC ASA and tiotropium.

- "Inappropriate compliance" for atenolol. Cause cannot be identified.

- "Wrong drug" caused by more effective drug therapy available for tiotropium.

- "Wrong drug" caused by contraindication present for atenolol in asthma.

5.2 Using the criteria provided, identify Mrs. Rifkin's drug therapy problems as serious, acute, both, or neither and prioritize the problems as Priority I, II or III.

Actual problems:

- "Adverse drug reaction" caused by undesirable effect caused by atenolol.

- "Dosage too low" caused by wrong dosage for calcium carbonate.

Potential problems:

- "Needs additional drug therapy" caused by need for synergistic therapy with calcium and a biphosphonate.

- "Wrong drug" caused by more effective drug therapy available for esomeprazole.

5.3 Reword each of these ill-defined goals to ones that are achievable, measurable, and consistent with the pharmacist's responsibilities.

a. Control the patient's migraine headaches.

b. The patient will receive smoking cessation education.

c. The patient will be evaluated for insertion of tympanostomy tubes.

5.4 Are these goals or plans? Why? If they are plans, reword them into goals.

a. Start the patient on enalapril 5 mg po qd for hypertension.

b. Change the medication from pravastatin 20 mg qd to atorvastatin 20 mg qd.

c. The patient will take his blood pressure at home twice weekly.

d. Enroll the patient in our asthma management program.

5.5 Below is the revised list of drug therapy problems for Mrs. Rifkin. For each drug therapy problem, write a compound goal. Remember to make each goal measurable, achievable, consistent with your responsibilities, and well defined.

a. Adverse effect of atenolol.

b. Dosage too low of calcium.

c. Needs additional drug therapy (calcium).

d. Wrong drug (esomeprazole).

5.6. List at least two options to resolve each of Mrs. Rifkin's drug therapy problems listed below.

a. Adverse effect of atenolol.

b. Dosage too low of calcium.

c. Needs additional drug therapy (calcium).

d. Wrong drug (esomeprazole).

5.7 Why is the care plan to discontinue atenolol a poor one to treat Mrs. Rifkin's atenolol-induced fatigue?

5.8 Develop a patient-focused intervention around the following drug therapy problems identified in Mrs. Rifkin:

• Fatigue as adverse effect of atenolol.

• Dosage too low of calcium carbonate.

5.9 Develop a specific, detailed drug-focused intervention around the following drug therapy problems identified in Mrs. Rifkin:

a. Adverse effect of atenolol of fatigue.

b. Dosage too low of calcium carbonate.

5.10 In question 5.6, possible interventions were developed for each of Mrs. Rifkin's drug therapy problems. Use these choices to create a care plan for each drug therapy problem. Your care plan should have the following characteristics:

- It should be patient-focused, drug-focused or both depending on patient needs.

- Given everything you know about the patient, the health care system, and drug therapy it should be the best choice of those available and you should justify your choice.

- It should be as specific as possible. What exactly must the patient and/or physician do? Specifically what therapy do you recommend?

- It should include verification that the patient has all necessary drugs and supplies and knows how to take/use them.

- It includes a clinically appropriate (subjective and objective information if clinically necessary) patient monitoring or follow-up plan that the patient understands and agrees to.

- It specifies who must monitor or follow up on what parameter and when.

1. Adverse effect of atenolol: fatigue.

   a. Decrease dose of atenolol to 25 mg qd;

   b. Change atenolol to chlorthalidone 25 mg po qd;

   c. Change atenolol to prazosin 1 mg qd.

2. Dosage too low of calcium.

   a. Increase calcium to calcium carbonate 1500 mg bid with meals;

   b. Change calcium to calcium citrate 950 mg 2 tablets tid with meals.

3. Needs additional drug therapy (calcium).

   a. Add alendronate 35 mg q weekly;

   b. Add risedronate 35 mg weekly;

   c. Add ibandronate 150 mg q monthly.

4. Wrong drug (esomeprazole).

   a. Change esomeprazole to generic omeprazole 20 mg qd;

   b. Change esomeprazole to lansoprazole 15 mg qd.

5.11 Write a letter to Dr. Hale, Mrs. Rifkin's physician. Your letter should describe what you have done, what drug therapy problems you have found, what you propose to do about them, your proposed monitoring plan and what (if anything) you want Dr. Hale to do. Make sure your letter is clear, concise (no more than 1 page), and does not include any wording or phrases that may offend Dr. Hale.

References

1. Kohn LT, Corrigan JM, Donaldson MS, eds. *To Err is Human: Building a Safer Health System*. Washington, DC: National Academy Press; 2000:26.

2. Aspden P, Wolcott J, Bootman JL, et al., eds. *Preventing Medication Errors: Quality Chasm Series Free Executive Summary*. Available at: http://www.nap.edu/catalog/11623.html. Accessed August 14, 2006.

Notes

Documentation 6

Jay D. Currie

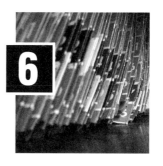

Documenting the pharmacist–patient encounter is a critical step in the pharmaceutical care process. Pharmacists must record their assessment and the actions they took or will take. This creates a valuable record for use in providing future care to the patient.

Without a written record, there is no proof that the pharmacist contributed to the care of the patient. Plus the process of producing documentation is an opportunity for the pharmacist to contemplate and re-evaluate the data collected and the care plan generated. No pharmacist is capable of remembering all the details regarding specific patients. And a good record of care is also useful for audits conducted by third-party payers and as legal evidence, should information about a patient's care ever be needed by the courts.

It is important to distinguish documentation of patient care from that of pharmacists' interventions or activities as they perform their clinical duties. The former involves the creation and use of a patient medical record, while the latter is a tool for use in recording and collating pharmacist contribution to patient care. Intervention documentation is a pharmacist-focused, not a patient-focused, process. Ultimately, the most useful documentation systems will be those which facilitate patient care, streamline billing for services delivered by the pharmacist, and allow for the collation of information on activities, effectiveness, and quality of care delivered.

Documentation occurs after data collection and evaluation, drug therapy problem-solving, and care plan development. Next to taking on new patient care responsibilities, maintaining a patient documentation system is the hardest task for pharmacists making the transition to pharmaceutical care. Most pharmacists have not previously engaged in extensive documentation of cognitive and care activities and have not developed the

In this chapter, the following concepts are reviewed:

- The importance of documentation in the care process.

- The difference between documentation of patient care and pharmacist intervention documentation.

- The relationship between the patient care process and documentation.

- Components of a patient care record.

- Components of a note documenting a patient care encounter.

- The concept of a problem-oriented pharmacy record.

- Components and structure of a SOAP note.

full set of skills necessary to complete these tasks. Like many other pharmaceutical care functions, creating useful and concise documentation requires a restructuring of the pharmacist's thought process.

As pharmacists become more patient care-oriented they will need to further refine their documentation skills. This process is not intuitive, as Becker et al. found that about one-fourth of pharmacist documentation examples submitted to qualify for participation in a state pharmaceutical care program did not include mention of actual or intended follow-up with the patient.[1]

More than Completing Forms

Documentation is much more than filling out forms during the patient interview. Data collection forms are helpful tools, but no ideal form is available for all patients and all situations. And, as mentioned in Chapter 3, pharmacists must guard against concentrating more on the form than on the patient. Instead they should take only enough notes to be able to reconstruct the patient encounter later. An exception would be when the pharmacist is entering detailed data (for example, blood pressure or pulse rate) directly onto a flow sheet that is a permanent part of the patient record.

Documentation is much more than filling out forms during the patient interview.

Each patient's entire record, as well as pertinent information and comments regarding a patient's therapy, should be readily retrievable. Other caregivers in the pharmacy or institution must be able to understand and use the records with no misunderstanding. In records that facilitate patient care, the following must be easily accessible:

• An accurate history of patient-related information.

• The thoughts and conclusions of the pharmacist.

• A current care plan.

• Instructions about what should take place during the next encounter to monitor the patient.

Activities completed by the pharmacist and the clinical outcomes related to those activities are included in this type of patient care documentation. Depending on the methods used, these measures may need to be abstracted from the record as the collation of pharmacist activities is not an intrinsic function of patient care documentation.

Types of Documentation Systems

Basic components of a patient record were outlined in the Omnibus Budget Reconciliation Act of 1990 (OBRA '90), a law that requires not only medication counseling for Medicaid patients but also the creation of records containing patient demographic information, a medication list, a listing of conditions or disease states, and comments on the patient's drug therapy. Although this type of record has been mandated since January 1993, the record-keeping systems in many pharmacies are not conducive to creating readily retrievable patient-specific information. Some pharmacists record comments on the back of the prescription order, which is a problem because its size limits the amount of information it can carry. Plus often it is filed away, never to be viewed again.

Depending on the practice setting, the pharmacist may have a free-standing patient record that they create and maintain, or they may be using a record that is shared by the various care providers in that practice location. Many pharmacists working in clinics or in health systems will be contributing to a patient record that is used by multiple providers with a variety of specialties. How the pharmacist will document the care they provide may be established by policies of the organization. In other cases the pharmacist will work with other providers to determine the most appropriate methodology.

As pharmacists begin to provide pharmaceutical care, they discover not only that they need an efficient documentation system but also how challenging it is to create one. Although phar-

"If we didn't document it, we didn't do it —or at least we can't prove it" is a common sentiment among pharmaceutical care practitioners.

TABLE 6-1

The Value of Documentation

Documentation has the following benefits:

- Provides a permanent record of patient information that the pharmacist has collected and analyzed, as well as of the patient's care plan.

- Efficiently communicates key information to colleagues at the practice site and to other health care providers.

- Contributes to a repository of accumulated patient data.

- Provides evidence of the pharmacist's actions and successes in patient care.

- Serves as a legal record of care provided.

- Provides back-up for billing requests and furnishes answers to questions from third-party payers.

macists often keep computer records related to prescription orders, those allowed by dispensing systems may be inadequate. Record-keeping portions of dispensing software often do not allow sufficient space for comments on the patient's drug therapy. Cryptic notes created to fit in tiny data fields can be more dangerous than helpful in caring for patients. While some necessary information can be stored in these records, they are not designed to thoroughly document the care provided.

Today several dispensing software programs include pharmaceutical care modules that provide an improved patient care documentation format. Other programs link their dispensing modules to available pharmaceutical care documentation programs. Freestanding programs are also available. Pharmacists should postpone decisions about buying a computerized documentation system until they have adequate experience in providing care and completing basic documentation. Which product or add-on is appropriate depends on the methods being used in providing patient care and the needs for documentation.

Issues to be considered in evaluating a documentation package are listed in Table 6-2. Pharmacists working in organizations with existing documentation systems are encouraged to include their documentation in that system to allow for better integration of care. Regardless of practice setting, exchange of patient-specific medication-related information between providers and between care settings is recommended for improving medication safety.[2]

A recently published survey of community pharmacists providing expanded patient care services attempted to identify characteristics of current documentation systems and characteristics of systems pharmacists desired in an ideal documentation system.[3] Over half of the respondents to the survey were using a paper documentation system, while 42% were using either a commercial or personally developed computer-based system. A majority of pharmacists using the paper system agreed to statements that it was of reasonable cost, added value to their practice, allowed for free-form text entry, met the needs of the practice site, and was easy to use. Although evaluating their systems as having cost-related considerations, pharmacists using computerized systems agreed with statements indicating their systems required less time, were easier to use, allowed for compact storage of information, and more easily retrieved patient information and generated reports. Pharmacists desired systems that would meet their needs to document all patient care services provided in the practice, were reasonably priced, were time efficient and easy to use, and would generate patient reports.

Pharmacists can begin providing care with a simple paper documentation system and then investigate more expensive systems after they have a better sense of what will work for them. Pharmacists joke that pharmaceutical care can be provided using only a Big Chief writing tablet and a crayon. While this is true, development of an efficient system for documentation is important for an efficient practice.

How sophisticated the initial paper system should be depends on how long it will be used. If the system will be temporary, inexpensive manila folders work well. If the system is likely to become a permanent part of patient care it may be worth investing in one like those in other professional practices, which code charts by color, letter, and date. In either type of paper system there must be a way to affix pages in the chart so that patient data are not lost or disorganized. Many pharmacies keep a "hard"

TABLE 6-2

Attributes to Consider in Documentation Programs

Pharmacists would be wise to put off investing in computerized documentation software until they have enough pharmaceutical care experience to know what they really need. Because the market is in flux and published information quickly becomes outdated, the best way to identify vendors is to contact the American Society for Automation in Pharmacy, 492 Norristown Rd., Suite 160, Blue Bell, PA 19422. Telephone: (610) 825-7783, Fax: (610) 825-7641. www.asapnet.org/

When looking for a computer documentation software package, consider these issues:

- Overall ease of use.
- Complexity of entry.
- Time required to learn the system.
- Speed of entry.
- Usefulness for collecting and documenting relevant information.
- Ease with which documentation tasks can be delegated to clerical staff.
- Quality of report generation.
- Billing capabilities.
- HIPAA compliance.
- Encryption and other privacy concerns if a web-based application.

- Hardware requirements.
- The system's flexibility and ability to be customized.
- Ease of integration with current software.
- Vendor responsiveness to user needs.
- Technical support required from the vendor to set up the system, as well as to customize or upgrade it.
- Actual support provided.
- Cost.
- How often the system must be upgraded.
- Cost of upgrades.
- Network and multi-user capability.

or paper copy in addition to an electronic copy of patient records, but over time this may change.

As more physician practices and health systems incorporate electronic medical records and electronic prescribing into practice, pharmacy documentation systems will need to have the capabilities to interface with these external systems. Pharmacists working in these settings should seek to incorporate their documentation into these existing systems.

Problem-Oriented Records

Experience gained from the medical community suggests that problem-oriented records are the most efficient and useful. Developed in the early 1960s by Lawrence Weed,[4,5] the problem-oriented approach to documentation streamlines the amount of reading that practitioners must do to update themselves on a patient's status. The patient's medical chart is organized by medical problem and contains structured notes about each problem. Providers can determine the current diagnostic, therapeutic, and monitoring plans at a glance rather than having to extract them out of unformatted "narrations" about the patient and the care provided.

In pharmacy practices, organizing charts by drug therapy problem is analogous to the medical chart being organized by medical problem.

In pharmacy practices, organizing charts by drug therapy problem is analogous to the medical chart being organized by medical problem. By writing structured notes about each drug therapy problem or closely related group of problems, pharmacists can quickly locate the most recent entry and read the portion of the note devoted to the current plan and follow-up schedule. This speeds the process of deciding what to do next and when to do it. If pharmacists need additional information to further understand the care plan, they can review other relevant sections of the record. Eliminating extraneous material about patients and their medical needs speeds both documentation and interpretation of information.

Problem-Oriented Pharmacy Records

A problem-oriented pharmacy record (POPR) should conform to the guidelines in Table 6-3, as well as to Figure 6-1 (see Tables 6-3 and 6-4 for descriptions of elements in the figure). It also should contain a problem list that briefly delineates the important information in the chart. The problem list serves as an index for the patient record and allows for efficient use. As shown in the sample problem list (Figure 6-2), the Pharmaceutical Care Data Sheet lists the patient's medical problems, medication allergies, current medications, and drug therapy problems.

FIGURE 6-1

Tool for Evaluation of Documentation

Please check whether or not each element is present.　　Case I.D._____

Essential patient encounter elements

Yes　No

- ☐ ☐ 1. Date of encounter
- ☐ ☐ 2. Patient date of birth
- ☐ ☐ 3. Patient identifier
- ☐ ☐ 4. Reason for the encounter
- ☐ ☐ 5. History of present illness
- ☐ ☐ 6. Relevant Rx/OTC/alternative medication history/compliance
- ☐ ☐ 7. Assessment
- ☐ ☐ 8. Plan(s)/Action(s) to correct problem(s)
  - ☐ No drug therapy problems identified
- ☐ ☐ 9. Monitoring plan/follow-up

Encounter elements to be included if relevant

Relevant　　Present

Yes　No　　Yes　No

- ☐ ☐ 　☐ ☐ 10. Past medical history
- ☐ ☐ 　☐ ☐ 11. Family history
- ☐ ☐ 　☐ ☐ 12. Social history
- ☐ ☐ 　☐ ☐ 13. Objective information

Essential patient record elements

Yes　No

- ☐ ☐ 1. Patient identifier
- ☐ ☐ 2. Pharmacist identifier
- ☐ ☐ 3. Patient sex
- ☐ ☐ 4. Contact information
- ☐ ☐ 5. Allergies/ADRs
- ☐ ☐ 6. Medical problem(s) current and past
- ☐ ☐ 7. Rx/OTC/alternative medication history
- ☐ ☐ 8. Payment method/economic situation

Record elements to be included if relevant

Relevant　　Present

Yes　No　　Yes　No

- ☐ ☐ 　☐ ☐ 9. Family history
- ☐ ☐ 　☐ ☐ 10. Social history
- ☐ ☐ 　☐ ☐ 11. Patient race
- ☐ ☐ 　☐ ☐ 12. Objective information
- ☐ ☐ 　☐ ☐ 13. Special needs of patient
- ☐ ☐ 　☐ ☐ 14. Nonmedication therapy

FIGURE 6-2

Pharmaceutical Care Data Sheet

Pharmaceutical Care Record		
Name *Mary Blythe*	DOB 7/10/67	Allergies *NKDA,* Dogs, Cats, Dust, Grass, Pollen*

Medical Problem List

Date		No.	Problem
Active	Resolved		
-12/01		A	*Depression*
?<2000		B	*Allergic Rhinitis*
		C	
		D	
		E	
		F	
		G	
		H	
		I	
		J	
		K	
		L	
		M	
		N	
		O	
		P	
		Q	
		R	
		S	

Medication List

Date		Prob#	Drug and Str.	Dose
Start	Stop			
-9/02		A	*Serzone 150 mg*	*BID*
-6/02		B&A	*Benadryl 25 mg*	*4HS*
-1/02		B	*Vancenase AQ*	*2 BID*
-6/02		B	*Afrin*	*2 BID*
?			*APAP*	*PRN HA*

Drug Therapy Problem List

Date		No.	Drug Therapy Problem with Description
Identified	Resolved		
12/29/02		1	*Inappropriate compliance - overuse of Afrin and underuse of Vancenase AQ*
12/29/02		2	*Adverse drug reaction - nasal congestion from overuse of Afrin*
12/29/02		3	*Adverse drug reaction - nasal congestion and hypotension possibly due to Serzone*
12/29/02		4	*Dosage too high - dose and duration of Benadryl*
		5	
		6	
		7	
		8	
		9	
		10	
		11	
		12	
		13	
		14	

Copyright 1994. Iowa Center for Pharmaceutical Care.

*NKDA: No known drug allergies.

The section on drug therapy problems should identify the type and provide sufficient detail about the medication and problem encountered to clarify the situation (i.e., undesirable effect: nausea from aspirin). For each problem contained on the list there should be a note, or a series of notes, in the body of the chart that includes the corresponding details.

The medical problem list should convey diagnoses rather than symptoms. Listing of multiple symptoms (polyuria, nocturia, polydipsia, polyphagia, blurred vision) rather than a diagnosis (diabetes mellitus) will clutter the record and make it more difficult to use. Additionally, a symptom can be caused by a drug therapy problem and these should not be confused with an underlying medical problem.

The medication list should include all medications as well as nonprescription and nontraditional remedies. This list can be difficult to develop but is a valuable addition to the patient information available to the health care team. If this list is available elsewhere in the patient record it may not need to be generated again.

Updating the Chart

Patients' charts are never complete until a patient dies or stops receiving care from a practice. Their contents and problem lists constantly change, and as the chart grows it becomes an increasingly accurate record. Because information should never be removed from the chart, mechanisms must be developed to allow for constant evolution. In the example on page 146, the "start" and "stop" columns in the "medication list" section are used to continually update the list without removing information.

If the list becomes unwieldy a new list can be created and dated to supersede the old one. During the transcription process it is important to check that information is being transferred accurately. The old list then goes behind the new one or into an archival portion of the chart. The new list becomes the only place to look for pertinent information on current problems.

Flow Sheets

Flow sheets are often included in patient charts to present data compactly. Weight, blood pressure, pulse, and other vital signs may be easier to follow if recorded in a table. Various doses of a drug, physical findings, and laboratory results may also be easier to track and analyze when presented in a table. Charting the values in a graph is another way to represent data in a readily interpretable way. Entire courses of disease management can often be documented for months or years on a single page of a well-designed flow sheet. An example of a flow sheet appears in Figure 6-3.

TABLE 6-3

Brief Descriptions of Essential Patient Record Elements

The following text explains the patient record elements in Figure 6-1:

1. **Patient identifier** (name, name code, or code number).

2. **Patient date of birth** or method to determine patient age.

3. **Patient sex** (male, female, or undetermined).

4. **Contact information.** Address, telephone number, etc. should be available and current in the chart. Indicate patient preference for method of contact.

5. **Allergies/ADRs.** Patient medication allergies and adverse drug reaction history or the lack thereof.

6. **Medical problem(s) current and past.** Descriptions of current versus remote problems should be clear, and relative dates of diagnosis or resolution of the diagnosis are included. Environmental allergies should be noted if relevant.

7. **Rx/OTC/alternative medication history.** A comprehensive listing including prescription, nonprescription, vitamin, herbal, and homeopathic treatments, with prescribed dose, actual regimen, adverse drug reaction history, and compliance noted.

8. **Payment method/economic situation.** Information on insurance carrier, coverage limitations, and patient identification number. Information on the patient's current economic situation that could affect treatment should be retrievable.

9. **Family history.** A listing of medical conditions of family members that relate to the health care of the patient.

10. **Social history.** A listing of social considerations that may relate to the health care situation, including tobacco, alcohol, or recreational drug use, and positive health-related habits.

11. **Patient race.**

12. **Objective information.** A compilation of testing results from the pharmacy practice or other testing site. Note if information is collected from other providers and include vital statistics such as height, weight, temperature, respiration, pulse, and blood pressure.

13. **Special needs of patient.** A listing of such things as visual or hearing impairment, need for assistive devices, special educational needs, etc., or a notation if there are no special needs.

14. **Nonmedication therapy.** Treatments, dietary regimens, physical activity or other therapy the patient is receiving that does not involve medications, plus a note if nonmedication therapies are not being used.

FIGURE 6-3

Pharmaceutical Care Flow Sheet

	DATES									
Test										

TABLE 6-4

Brief Descriptions of Essential Patient Encounter Elements

The essential elements in Figure 6-1 may be present in the chart and referred to in the note, but not repeated in the encounter note itself.

If the documentation pertains to a follow-up encounter, the note should include similar elements as described, but could be abbreviated, with some elements unnecessary if they are contained in the original encounter note.

1. **Date of encounter.** Date of the pharmacist encounter with the patient.

2. **Pharmacist identifier.** Clear identification of the pharmacist providing care to the patient.

3. **Patient identifier.** The patient can be identified by name, name code, or code number.

4. **Reason for the encounter.** The reason for the interaction with the patient can be identified. This could be initiated by patient, pharmacist, or other health care provider. This could be the chief complaint if the patient initiated the interaction with a new problem, the consult request from another provider or caregiver, or through drug regimen review if pharmacist-initiated.

5. **History of present illness.** An adequate description exists of the relevant events leading up to the encounter. This could include the source of the information (patient, caregiver, clinical record), description of the complaint, significant positive and negative information on the quality, severity, duration, time variation, modifying factors or associated symptoms. If a follow-up encounter, progress toward meeting established goals should be included.

6. **Relevant Rx/OTC/alternative medication history/compliance.** A listing of medications, regimens, allergies, recent changes or other information pertaining to the presenting problem. This should include prescription, nonprescription, vitamin, herbal and homeopathic treatments. If medications are taken, compliance should be addressed. If there is no relevant medication history this should also be noted.

7. **Assessment.** Conclusions reached by the pharmacist after assessment of the drug therapy. A clear statement of the drug therapy problem, if identified, and its current status should be mentioned. Professional judgement as to the credibility of the information collected may be stated.

8. **Plan(s)/Action(s) to correct problem(s).** A listing of planned steps to achieve the goals established with the patient for the patient's drug therapy. May be planned interventions or actions already taken, such as discussions with or recommendations made to the patient, caregiver or other health care provider, or referrals made to other health care providers. It should distinguish what has been completed from what is contemplated or planned for the future. Plans may address patient understanding of the problem and plan. Plan should address each recommendation with specific implementation steps. The goal of the therapy should be implicitly or explicitly stated.

9. **Monitoring plan/follow-up.** Steps to monitor the outcomes of actions taken. These should include both the components to be monitored and a schedule for that monitoring. A statement should be included as to the date or time span until the next monitoring encounter, including the method of conducting that encounter (i.e., telephone call, in-store contact, etc.) It should be clear if the follow-up will be initiated by the pharmacist, patient, or other health care provider.

TABLE 6-4

Brief Descriptions of Essential Patient Encounter Elements, continued

10. **Past medical history.** A listing of disease states or other complaints that affect the problem for the current encounter including prior testing or evaluation, using appropriate detail.

11. **Family history.** Modifying factors of the current situation regarding medical problems in the patient's family should be listed when pertinent to the disease state or medications.

12. **Social history.** Other modifying factors, such as diet, alcohol, tobacco, other recreational drug use, caregiver status and occupation, that can affect therapy should be included if relevant.

13. **Objective information.** Objective information considered in the evaluation should be included. This might include vital signs, laboratory results, diagnostic signs or physical examination results.

Other Sections

Depending on the particular practice, the patient population, and the information collected, other sections may be necessary in the chart. For example, a separate section for laboratory reports may be needed so the provider does not have to sift through the whole chart to find them. Another section might contain records generated outside the pharmacy, such as hospitalization reports, pre-admission pharmacy records, physician records, and public or home health nursing reports.

Correspondence, both incoming and outgoing, can make up another section. The correspondence section might include letters or faxes to and from physicians, other health care providers, caregivers, or insurance companies. It also could include a copy of the release to share correspondence signed by the patient or legal representative. Requirements vary according to the individual practice; it is up to each pharmacy to decide what to include in the chart.

Pharmacists should stay abreast of the ultimate rules developed for the implementation of the Health Insurance Portability and Accountability Act of 1996 (HIPAA). These rules may mandate additional record-keeping needs to assure the confidentiality and privacy of the patient's pharmacy record.

Problem-Oriented Content

Problem-oriented notes form the substance of the patient chart. These notes tell the pharmacist or other providers what information was considered in evaluating the patient's drug therapy, how the data were evaluated, details of the care plan, steps taken to date to implement the plan, outcome measures to be assessed, and the schedule for completing outcome assessments.

Each note is written about a single problem, or about a closely related group of problems, regarding the disease state, medication, or drug-related problem involved. The problems "inappropriate duration-5-day treatment with penicillin for strep throat" and "undesirable effect-constipation due to iron supplementation" identified at a single patient encounter would best be handled with two separate notes, because they are unrelated. In contrast, the problems "inappropriate duration-5-day treatment with penicillin for strep throat" and "need for additional drug therapy-untreated pain due to strep throat" are related and could be efficiently documented in one note.

Any two or more notes that would have a majority of the subjective and objective information duplicated would be candidates for being combined into one note. If the patient assessment reveals no drug therapy problems, a note stating that should

---

TABLE 6-5

Guidelines for Patient Charts

- The pharmacy record should include all the important demographic and historical information about the patient as well as details about ongoing care.

- All sheets should be identified by patient name or identification number in case they become separated from the chart. Information entered into a permanent patient record should never be removed.

- Maintain one complete record for each patient. Generating separate records for different purposes is not only redundant and time consuming, but also tremendously inefficient because it means that multiple records must be consulted.

- The record should be updated each time the pharmacist interacts with the patient, or whenever there is additional information on the patient.

- Be sure abbreviations or other documentation shortcuts are clear. Standard medical abbreviations are listed in a number of reference books.

- Some pharmacists dictate their notes for patient records into a tape recorder for transcription. When errors are found during review of transcribed or handwritten notes, or if changes are made for any reason, the original text should be retained in readable form (not crossed or opaqued out). Put a single line through the error, write in the correction, and initial it. If simple editing is insufficient an addendum should be used for clarification. Once the note is signed by the care provider who generated it, no changes should be made to the note.

- Patient records should never be destroyed. If patients become "inactive" and stop using the pharmacy their charts may be removed from the active files and archived. Pharmacists can find out the requirements in their state for maintaining records and the statute of limitations for lawsuits by checking with their liability insurance provider or the state board of pharmacy.

be included, and should contain the information leading to that conclusion and the plans for future re-evaluation of the patient.

Each note should be dated and if multiple entries are made on the same day, record the time of each. Each note should also be titled, usually by using the drug-related problem discussed in the note. This title should be the same as that used on the problem list so these are clearly linked in the record. If more than one problem is covered in a note, all of them should be included in the title.

Documenting the drug therapy problem (either in the note's title or as the assessment) serves as a safeguard for pharmacists. Using the taxonomy of drug therapy problems provides evidence that they are working within the scope of pharmacy practice.

Some pharmacists may prefer to title a note with the medical problem it discusses, especially if they regularly share records with physicians or other health care professionals who are accustomed to the medical problem format. If the organization where the pharmacist works is using an electronic medical record it might be required that notes are linked through this mechanism. Other pharmacists may want to title the note with the medication involved. The way the notes are titled is less important than using a consistent approach and including the necessary information.

TABLE 6-6

A Sampling of Paper Chart Suppliers

Here is a short list of vendors that supply paper charting systems.

Bibbero Systems, Inc. 1300 N. McDowell Blvd. Petaluma, CA 94954-1180 800-242-2376 www.bibbero.com	Ames Color-File 12 Tyler Street; P.O. Box 120 Somerville, MA 02143-0120 800-343-2040 www.amescolorfile.com/
Safeguard Business Systems, Inc. 8585 N. Stemmons Freeway, Suite 600 N Dallas, Texas 75247 800-336-0636 www.gosafeguard.com	Tab US Headquarters 605 Fourth Street Mayville, WI 53050 888-466-8228 www.tab.com

Contents of a Note

The notes in the chart should be structured in a consistent format to promote efficient use in the delivery of care and assist the pharmacist in providing future care to the patient. A number of methods for documentation of pharmacist activities have been proposed,[6,7] along with the widely used SOAP note, described on page 155. The actual method or format used to document care is not as important as the contents of the record. Style and format should also take into account health care organization norms and whether or not the note will be used by other health care providers.

In an effort to define necessary components to be included in a pharmacist note, Currie et al. published guidelines on the information to be included both in a record of care for an individual encounter with a patient and in a more comprehensive record (the patient chart) for a patient receiving ongoing care.[8] These guidelines were developed using practitioner and expert panel input that included pharmacists from community, hospital, managed care, academic, and clinical practice settings as well as other health professionals from the quality assessment, nursing, and medical professions.

The authors report the product of a consensus development process designed to identify the components that must be present in a record of care to allow that record to be judged on the quality of the care provided. This team developed the Tool for Evaluation of Documentation, or TED, that can be used by pharmacists or organizations to judge the completeness of pharmacists' documentation and thus assess the quality of the care provided. (See Figure 6-1 and Tables 6-3 and 6-4 for the TED and an explanation of its components.) This tool can be used to assess a note written by a pharmacist no matter what the format or method of documentation. Pharmacists will find the form to be a useful reference as they are learning to write notes, assessing the quality of their own notes, and implementing quality assurance methods in their practice.

As pharmacists develop proficiency at note writing (including all the necessary elements in the documentation of care) they can begin concentrating on the quality of the information included. Writing notes repeatedly using the same format and structure will allow development of efficiency in completing the documentation. Eventually the writer will be able to consider only the information going into the note as they are writing or dictating. Getting feedback from colleagues on what was communicated to them will help pharmacists refine their note writing skills, as will providing future care based on their notes.

SOAP Notes

The SOAP format is widely used in health care, as it is easily read and comprehended by other health care professionals. SOAP is an acronym that stands for Subjective, Objective, Assessment, and Plan. Each term relates to a section of the note that contains a specific type of information. They directly relate to the data collection, problem identification, and problem-solving steps discussed in previous chapters. Because the note structure corresponds to the care process completed with the patient it makes for a logical documentation method. Developing a consistent approach to writing these notes helps pharmacists provide efficient care to patients. Summarizing patient information in this format is a useful tool when discussing patients with other health care providers.

SOAP is an acronym that stands for Subjective, Objective, Assessment, and Plan.

The subjective and objective portions of the documentation contain information from the patient, exams performed, and laboratory or other tests performed on the patient. The information taken into account as patient's problems are considered and how pharmacists decide to resolve it should also be included. For example, if the pharmacist recommended a drug that is available generically because the patient stated that he couldn't afford expensive treatment, include that in the subjective portion of the note. If he recommended a lower dose of a renally-eliminated drug because the patient has evidence of decreased renal function, that should be included in the objective section.

Subjective and objective information serve as the basis for the assessment and treatment plan. When following up about a problem, these sections describe the interim and current status of patients. Both the assessment and the plan should convey what the provider believed was going on with the patient, what was done on that date, and follow-up.

Subjective Information

The subjective section of the note is for recording information obtained from the patient or caregiver, as well as historical information that may not be known objectively. Only information pertinent to specific drug therapy problems should be included. Material that should go in this section includes:

• Patient's chief complaint or reason for the patient encounter.

• Patient's history of present illness (HPI).

• Past medical history (PMH).

- Social or family history (SH or FH).

- Allergies.

- Previous adverse drug reactions (ADR).

- Review of systems (ROS).

This section should also specify the medications involved and explain how the patient is taking them. Practitioners sometimes disagree about where the medication history should be recorded. If what the pharmacist is getting from the patient is undocumented history it might fit under the subjective heading. Or he may feel he has objective knowledge of the patient's regimen based on dispensing or medication administration record. What is essential is documenting the patient's history in either the subjective or objective section of the note, along with the other information collected about the patient.

Objective Information

The objective part of the note is used to document data such as:

- Vital signs.

- Laboratory test results (from the original tests, not patient history).

- Findings from other tests.

- Physical examination results from a trained examiner.

BOX 6-1

Confidentiality

Confidentiality of the patient's pharmacy records must be guarded carefully. Within the pharmacy, a system should be in place to ensure the security of patient records, whether they are computerized or on paper. Firm policies should govern which pharmacy employees have access to patient charts, and in what capacity.

The pharmacists and the pharmacy staff must understand that information in the record is to be provided to others only when authorized by the patient in writing (see the Authorization to Release Medical Information form, Figure 3-7) or when required by law. The confidentiality issue is especially important as pharmacists seek payment for services through third-party payers. Following HIPAA rules on information collection, storage, sharing, and transmission is essential.

Indicating who generated the objective data (and including the date) may be appropriate. For example: "Physical exam 12/20/06 by Dr. Smith indicated HEENT [head, eyes, ears, nose, and throat] exam WNL [within normal limits]."

The Assessment

The assessment part of the note allows pharmacists to document what they feel is the current status of the patient's problems. The assessment should be based on data contained in the subjective and objective sections. It will pertain to the title of the note but will elaborate on the problems rather than simply restating them. If the note is untitled, then pharmacists must be sure to explicitly state the drug therapy problem in this section of the note.

When a problem is first identified, the pharmacist may enter a brief description followed by the words "newly identified." When an assessment note is written after re-evaluating a problem, such as after a follow-up call, use terms such as "resolved" or "worsened" to indicate the status of the problem. The assessment section is a good place to document special considerations or the rationale for the care plan if stating the reason for the assessment seems necessary.

The Plan

The plan section is a record of what a pharmacist did or plans to do for the patient, such as providing patient education or making recommendations to the patient, physician, or caregiver. The recommendations and how they will be implemented should be clear to the reader. It should also be obvious whether the action has already been taken or is still being considered.

The pharmacist may want to separate the part of the plan that discusses action taken or anticipated from the portion that indicates how outcomes will be monitored. Physicians often separate their plans into diagnostic (Dx), therapeutic (Tx), and follow-up (F/U); pharmacists may wish to do the same by including a subsection on follow-up.

Follow-up is an important part of the plan, and it should be documented. In practice this is a step that is often neglected—possibly a carry-over from pharmacists in the past not assuming responsibility for the outcomes. This must be changed.[1] In his book *Knowledge Coupling: New Premises and New Tools for Medical Care and Education*, Lawrence Weed discusses the importance of developing a mechanism for following up each problem identified.[9] A quote from the book follows:

"Faulty understanding and defective decisions may be expected at the outset of a new case. Indeed, they are inevitable in the face of multiple variables. But failure to follow up rigorously the results of those decisions is inexcusable. Action without follow-up is arrogance, especially where the objects of that action are living systems about which nothing is completely understood and in which conditions never remain fixed."

The F/U section of the plan should include the interval planned before follow-up is necessary, contact information as necessary, the monitoring parameters that will be assessed, and what will be done with data. Here is an example:

• F/U: Call patient at home in 3 weeks, assess ibuprofen effectiveness in relief of arthritis symptoms (pain < 3/10), any nausea/dyspepsia, changes in stool color. If arthritis improved and no ADR, would continue at present dose, F/U again in 1 month. If no apparent ADR and Sx [symptoms] not relieved would call Dr. and recommend dosage increase to ibuprofen 600 mg QID [four times daily]. If ADR consider different dose or drug.

After the SOAP note is written, it should be signed by the author (the provider giving the care documented in the note).

In this example contingency plans are included as they were developed, so they will not need to be thought through again at the time of follow-up. The pharmacist should be able to read the plan and know exactly what happened and what is intended next. Furthermore, a colleague should be able to read, interpret, and act on the plan if the recording pharmacist is not available.

The desired therapeutic outcome (relief of arthritis symptoms) and possible negative outcomes that are anticipated (nausea/dyspepsia, changes in stool color) are appropriate to be placed in the follow-up part of the plan because these are parameters to be monitored. Plus the follow-up section is often the best place to document the patient's therapeutic goals (decrease symptom of pain to < 3/10) since the pharmacist will determine whether those goals have been met.

New Notes for New Problems

After the SOAP note is written, it should be signed by the author (the provider giving the care documented in the note). When the patient receives subsequent care, a new SOAP note should be generated for each problem. This is a better approach than attaching addenda to previously generated notes. Follow-up notes are often short, and only need to cover changes and developments occurring between care episodes. Using a consistent format for the notes promotes efficiency as well as easier interpretation of the record by others, including physicians. Adhering to a standard format also helps pharmacists to quickly locate data they wish to present to patients and health care providers, thus saving time and subtly underscoring the pharmacist's professionalism. Whether or not the SOAP format is used, documentation of necessary information and creation of a patient record are essential to providing quality care to patients.

The pharmacist's ability to write SOAP notes or notes in another format, and to keep good records, improves with practice. Providing quality care and documenting it for all to see brings pharmacists one step closer to being integral members of the health care team.

Examples of documentation are given with each case discussed in Chapters 7-10.

Self Assessment Questions

6.1 List the functions of patient care documentation.

6.2 How does documentation of care differ from completing forms during the interview process?

6.3 What are the basic components of a problem-oriented patient record?

6.4 How does the documentation in a SOAP note parallel the care process?

6.5 Restructure the following story, written by pharmacist Joe Martin, into a SOAP note:

Jane came into the pharmacy today to get her Imitrex 100 mg tablets refilled again. She said she was having to use three tablets per day to treat her headaches. I told her not to do this as it was too much. She is only supposed to take a maximum of two tablets per day. She said she stopped the propranolol 20 mg twice daily she was taking about two weeks ago as she didn't think it helped anymore. I called the doctor to recommend desipramine 25 mg at HS for prophylaxis. I told her she should to talk with her physician before she stopped that because that can make her headaches worse as well. She says she will try to cut back on her use of the

Imitrex, but doesn't know about starting back on the propranolol as it made her have nightmares. I told her I would follow-up with her in one week to see how it was going. I checked her refills and I believe she is taking what she says.

6.6 Why is documenting the follow-up with a patient important?

Reflection Question

Think about a pharmacy practice you have seen or have worked in. How do pharmacists document the care they provide to patients beyond completion of the prescription filling process? Do they document differently if the care involves nonprescription medications, prescription medications, or other care services?

References

1. Becker C, Bjornson DC, Kuhle JW. Pharmacist care plans and documentation of follow-up before the Iowa pharmaceutical case management program. *J Am Pharm Assoc.* 2004;44(3):350-7.

2. Aspden P, Wolcott J, Bootman JL, et al., eds. Committee on Identifying and Preventing Medication Errors. *Preventing Medication Errors: Quality Chasm Series.* Washington, DC: National Academy Press; 2006. Executive Summary available online at http://newton.nap.edu/execsumm_pdf/11623. Accessed August 30, 2006.

3. Brock KA, Casper KA, Green TR, et al. Documentation of patient care services in a community pharmacy setting. *J Am Pharm Assoc.* 2006;46:378-84.

4. Weed LL. Medical records that guide and teach. *N Engl J Med.* 1968;278:593-600.

5. Weed LL. Medical records that guide and teach. *N Engl J Med.* 1968;278:652-7.

6. Strand LM, Cipolle RJ, Morley PC. Documenting the clinical pharmacist's activities: back to basics. *Drug Intell Clin Pharm.* 1988;22:63-7.

7. Canaday B, Yarborough P. Documenting pharmaceutical care: creating a standard. *Ann Pharmacother.* 1994;28:1292-6.

8. Currie JD, Doucette WR, Kuhle J, et al. Identification of essential elements in the documentation of pharmacist-provided care. *J Am Pharm Assoc.* 2002;43:41-9.

9. Weed LL. *Knowledge Coupling: New Premises and New Tools for Medical Care and Education.* New York: Springer-Verlag; 1994:115.

Part II
Skill Application in Practice

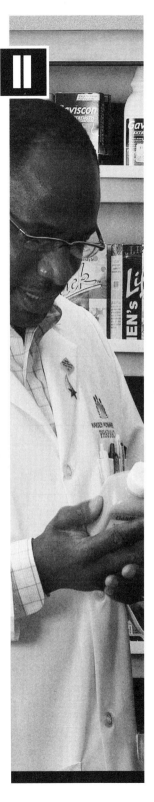

Part II of this book consists of four chapters that let you practice the pharmaceutical care skills described in Part I. The chapters highlight various practice settings, including community pharmacy, hospital inpatient, long-term-care, and ambulatory care clinic. Each chapter will give you the opportunity to apply all aspects of the patient care process.

Patient Case Studies

In these chapters you will complete the steps of the pharmaceutical care process using patient case studies developed for each of the four practice settings. For each case, your tasks will include deciding what information you need to collect, organizing it, analyzing it, and determining if it belongs in the comprehensive history.

You may also wish to consider how the information you decide to collect will help you care for the patient. If you are not sure what you would do with a piece of data, you will need to determine its importance and how it impacts the case. After deciding on the items required, you can use the comprehensive history (provided for each patient) to identify and prioritize drug therapy problems, create and implement a care plan, and document your patient care activities.

Applying these patient care skills in various practice settings will let you go through the processes repeatedly until they become natural. In addition, visualizing different environments for practicing pharmaceutical care allows you to consider some of the many opportunities available for pharmacists today.

Applying Clinical Skills in Community Pharmacies

Jay D. Currie

This chapter discusses the specifics of practicing pharmaceutical care in community pharmacies, and the cases at the end of the chapter test the patient care skills you need in those settings. More pharmacists work in community pharmacy than in any other type of practice.

However, practices described as "community" ones vary widely. They can be independently owned with one location or part of privately or publicly owned chains. They can be small or large. Some practices offer only professional services, and others handle a wide variety of products. Practices can focus on providing care and have space dedicated to that end, or they may focus on product distribution and offer little in the way of patient care facilities.

An increased focus on quality and safety in medication use, along with other Medication Therapy Management Service (MTMS) strategies, are likely to result in significant changes in community pharmacy practice over the next several years.

Most medications are delivered to patients in the community pharmacy setting. Therefore, this type of practice provides the greatest potential for interaction between pharmacists and the patients they care for. Although being in community practice is a great opportunity for pharmacists, most of them have traditionally focused on distribution of product and the provision of counseling mandated by the Omnibus Budget Reconciliation Act of 1990 (OBRA '90). They have also provided advice about nonprescription medications and other health-related questions. Pharmacists working in these settings are often physically remote from other health care providers and prescribers.

Now pharmacists are beginning to offer care-related services from their community pharmacy sites. These may be isolated services such as influenza immunization or screenings for dis-

More pharmacists work in community pharmacies than in any other type of practice.

eases like diabetes, hypertension, hyperlipidemia, or osteoporosis. Alternatively, they may offer services that are similar to those offered in ambulatory care pharmacy practices (see Chapter 10). The latter are usually done in partnership with another health provider, utilizing collaborative practice rules established for that state. Services generally develop from a patient need identified within the practice, often from experiences the pharmacist has in addressing drug therapy problems during the course of providing services related to drug distribution.

Community pharmacists are also looking for new ways to interact with patients and improve the outcomes of drug therapy. Innovative pharmacists have contracted with employers to provide health management and disease prevention services to their businesses. These arrangements, similar to the Asheville Project mentioned in Chapter 1, can benefit employers as they seek to keep their health care costs from escalating.

Community pharmacists have provided MTMS to high-risk patients in a number of states for several years. The continued growth in the delivery of these services is evolving as a function of Medicare Part D. As pharmacists show they can positively impact quality of care received by patients and overall health care costs, the delivery of this type of care will undoubtedly increase.

While the community setting offers wide access to patients, some barriers may limit the extent or quality of pharmacist–patient interactions. Many pharmacies are not designed with adequate patient counseling areas or other physical amenities which facilitate care. If there is no space the patient perceives as private, or no area where the pharmacist and patient can sit down together, the opportunities for interaction at the depth and to the extent needed to provide care are limited. Or if the practice environment does not support pharmaceutical care, the pharmacist may not have time to collect necessary information from patients as a part of routine daily functions. Organizational expectations of pharmacist activities and production measures need to be consistent with the provision of care. The pace of practice in some community pharmacies, which often must fill a large number of prescriptions to remain financially viable, is also an impediment.

Community pharmacists are often isolated from other providers, so they may collect their information directly from the patient or the patient's caregiver. Some limited laboratory or physical examination results might be available to the community pharmacist if they perform these themselves. Information can be obtained from outside providers, but this is often a multi-step process of faxing releases and requests with a resultant delay in gaining access to the information.

The care record used by the community pharmacist is likely one she develops and maintains on her own. Depending on the dispensing computer system used, the care record may be a separate paper or computer record, which limits the seamless transition between dispensing and care provision.

These deficiencies often decrease the efficiency of practice in the community setting. Pharmacists must anticipate that some of these obstacles to care will affect their practice and address them with a problem-solving approach. Programs and materials to assist in advancing practice are available to pharmacists through a variety of sources, including *A Practical Guide to Pharmaceutical Care,* Second Edition.

Self Assessment: Patient Case Studies

Use the following patient case studies to answer these questions.

1. After reading just the one-paragraph summary of each case, what additional information do you want to collect? What will be the source of that information?

2. Based on the comprehensive case history provided, identify and prioritize any drug therapy problems you find. Is each drug therapy problem actual or potential?

3. Determine a goal for each drug therapy problem.

4. Identify at least two ways to resolve/prevent each drug therapy problem.

5. Choose the best option, justify your choice, and create a care plan. Your care plan should include monitoring and follow-up parameters.

6. Determine how you will implement your care plan.

7. Write a SOAP note to document your patient care activities.

Patient: Sally Strathclyde

Sally presents to the pharmacy requesting refills on her asthma inhalers. A pharmacy technician takes the request and begins to process the refills, then calls you over with a question. She has noticed that Sally has an Advair and an albuterol inhaler prescribed by one physician along with a Serevent and an Azmacort inhaler prescribed by another physician. The tech asks you how to proceed.

Sally Strathclyde Case History
• **Chief Complaint:** Patient is a 36-year-old female who stopped into the pharmacy to get refills on her asthma inhalers.

• **History of Present Illness:** The patient has a history of asthma and has received treatment since childhood. She was on theophylline and cromolyn in the distant past before starting on inhaled steroids. Dr. Jones is her primary physician, but she sees two doctors in the same practice. On file, she has Advair and albuterol prescribed by one physician along with Serevent and Azmacort prescribed by another. She has received all these medications before, but never all four on the same day.

She has been using the Advair, Serevent, and Azmacort inhalers routinely on a daily basis, and she uses the albuterol inhaler about once per month. She used them all because she was confused about which inhaler was which. She was able to identify them only by color and was not familiar with their names. She evaluates her asthma control as very good.

• **Past Medication History:** Asthma since childhood

• **Medication List:**
Advair 250/50 mcg 1 puff BID.
Albuterol 2 puffs Q4H prn.
Serevent 1 puff BID.
Azmacort 4 puffs BID.

Patient: James Olson

James has come in to have his fasting lipid panel checked. (He learned you offered this service a month ago and made the appointment.) He has been a patient in your pharmacy for several years but has never received any lipid-lowering drugs there. He routinely gets lisinopril 10 mg once daily and Toprol XL 50 mg once daily for the treatment of hypertension.

James Olson Case History

- **Chief Complaint:** Cholesterol check per appointment.

- **History of Present Illness:** Patient is a 51-year-old WM here today in the pharmacy for a check of his cholesterol. Patient was last seen in Dr. Jones' office 9 months ago for lab work-up. At that time, doctor initiated lifestyle modifications in an attempt to reduce his cholesterol. Patient does not have the cholesterol results with him today, but states they were "high." Patient states that his next appointment is "not for a while." He appears to be very concerned about his high risk for a coronary event based on his family history and wants to know his progress.

  Patient stated that he has been willing to go to great lengths to stay off medication, but thinks he is doing about all he can do at present. He has been successful in decreasing salt and fat from his diet and eating more fish and chicken rather than red meat. Patient states that he has been successful in reducing the amount he smokes, has been "cutting down" and is currently at 3 cigarettes per day. He currently has a plan to quit "within the month." Patient states that he walks on a treadmill for 30 minutes 2 days per week and thinks he can double this to 4 days per week, although has tried unsuccessfully to do this in the past.

- **Past Medication History:**
  Hypertension x 3 years.
  Hyperlipidemia x 9 months.

- **Social History:** Patient is the owner of a small business. He currently smokes 3 cigarettes daily, with a 1-ppd history x 30 years. Patient drinks only decaffeinated coffee and denies any alcohol intake.

- **Family History:** Father had MI at age 57. Father's brother died of MI at age 37.

- **Medication List:**
  Lisinopril 10 mg 1 daily.
  Toprol XL 50 mg 1 daily.

- **Vitals:** Blood Pressure and Pulse.
  8/6/this year 140/100; pulse 70.
  7/5/this year 144/102, pulse 68.
  6/15/this year 140/104, pulse 72.

- **Laboratory:**
  8/6/06-Fasting.
  TC 209; HDL 33; LDL 150; TG 133; TC/HDL 6.4.
  FBG 94.

Notes

Applying Clinical Skills in Hospitals 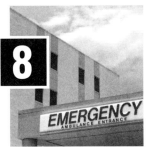 8
John P. Rovers

T his chapter discusses the specifics of practicing pharmaceutical care in hospitals. The cases at the end of the chapter
require you to test your care skills in inpatient settings.
Although pharmacists who work in these settings are typically
called hospital (or health system) pharmacists, such a simple de-
scriptor probably does not fully capture the diversity of practice
models and professional activities involved.

Decentralized hospital pharmacists may be assigned to a specific nursing unit and provide a blend of drug distribution and
clinical services. Or pharmacists may work in the central pharmacy, where their primary responsibility is managing drug distribution services while also providing clinical services to one or
more nursing units. Still others are full-time clinicians who typically have advanced training in an area of specialty practice (e.g.,
infectious diseases, critical care, or transplant, among others).
These specialty pharmacists are often full members of a medical
or surgical team and work closely with the team's physicians,
nurses, dieticians, and other practitioners to provide high quality clinical services. They may also provide consultation services,
upon request, to patients admitted to other nursing units.

Several clinical services are commonly provided no matter
what the practice model.[1] Many of these services are consistent with providing pharmaceutical care, but may require some
modifications to be fully compatible with a more patient-centered focus.

Drug therapy monitoring can be practiced in any inpatient
setting. The goal is to ensure that the patient is receiving the
safest, most effective, and most cost-effective medication available. This is generally done through the pharmacist screening
medication profiles to look for evidence that a patient's drug
therapy may not be optimal.

A pharmacist who monitors drug therapy has multiple opportunities to work directly with patients, nurses, and physicians to provide pharmaceutical care. As she screens patients' profiles and identifies potential issues related to drug safety or efficacy, she can discuss matters directly with the patient to obtain additional patient data and evaluate if one or more drug therapy problems is present.

Many inpatient pharmacists provide medication education to nurses, physicians, and patients. This may be done formally during in-service education sessions, informally during daily patient care rounds, or while conducting admission or discharge medication counseling sessions. The opportunity to speak with patients about their medications one-on-one presents the hospital pharmacist with an excellent opportunity to gather some patient history and evaluate the patient for any drug therapy problems.

Adverse drug reaction monitoring is often treated as a quality assurance activity. However, by speaking directly with patients who have suffered a possible reaction, the hospital pharmacist can further identify drug therapy problems related to the adverse effect.

Medication reconciliation pharmacists work to ensure that hospital providers have access to complete and accurate lists of patients' medications at all phases of the hospital stay (including admission, transfer between care units, and discharge). Any discrepancies between what a provider believes the patient is taking and what he is actually taking must be resolved. As discussed in Chapter 2, medication reconciliation pharmacists who take the time to talk with patients about their medication to uncover possible drug therapy problems can readily improve on the basic practice to encompass pharmaceutical care.

No matter what type of hospital pharmacy you practice or what nursing unit or medical team you may be assigned to, there are several factors that can influence the practice of pharmaceutical care in the inpatient setting. Some of these factors are helpful, while others are less so.

Helpful factors include the ready availability of both hospital personnel and patient care data. Since a patient's nurse is usually easy to find and speak with, being able to ask questions about the patient or communicate concerns about drug therapy is usually quite easy. Although physicians may not be as readily available, hospital pharmacists usually find that communication with them is often less difficult than it is for community pharmacists. Phar-

A pharmacist who monitors drug therapy has multiple opportunities to work directly with patients, nurses, and physicians to provide pharmaceutical care.

macists can page physicians who work full time in the hospital. Even with office-based physicians, most hospital pharmacists find it much easier to get through the various barriers and actually get the doctor on the phone. With both physicians and nurses, in-person or telephone communications are common and convenient. However, both nurses and physicians are busy, so these communications must be brief, well organized, and tightly focused.

Hospital pharmacists may document their activities in the patient's chart. Often, the written communication serves primarily to demonstrate that a service was provided or that a recommendation was made instead of being the primary means of communication with another provider.

Another helpful factor is the amount of patient-specific information available to the hospital pharmacist. A patient's chart contains a complete and current record of most of the information a pharmacist needs to make patient care decisions. A full medical history and physical examination, all laboratory and radiological investigations, consultation reports from other services, and the daily progress notes from a variety of providers give the pharmacist a plethora of useful clinical information. Not all of this information will be relevant, so pharmacists must often sort out useful from not useful information. Because little chart information is specifically drug-related, pharmacists must often gather additional information from the patient in order to identify drug therapy problems. In addition to the chart, patients' family members can often provide useful insights into the patient, his health, and his medication use. Family members are especially valuable resources for patients who cannot speak for themselves due to either illness or age.

Medication reconciliation pharmacists work to ensure that hospital providers have access to complete and accurate lists of patients' medications at all phases of the hospital stay (including admission, transfer between care units, and discharge).

Some features of hospital practice make pharmaceutical care a challenge. Since most patients are only in the hospital for 3 or 4 days, simply having time to meet with every patient to discuss drug therapy can be hard. Pharmacists may need to develop screening tools or other qualifying mechanisms to determine which patients should receive a pharmaceutical care work-up (e.g., patients taking warfarin or those taking more than five medications). Ideally, a pharmacist should visit with each of her patients daily since this allows for the greatest continuity of pharmaceutical care. Unfortunately, time constraints often make this difficult and care may be more episodic than daily. The short duration of stay can also make it a challenge to coordinate care with other pharmacists upon discharge.

Although nurses and physicians are easier to find and communicate with in a hospital, the nature of the communication can sometimes be trying. Pharmacists, nurses, physicians, and other health care professionals have different opinions about what their roles are in providing patient care and what they expect from other providers. Often, the hardest part about practicing pharmaceutical care in the inpatient setting is negotiating with everybody else on the health care team to see who is responsible for what and under which circumstances.

Clearly, inpatient practice has its own unique rewards and challenges to the practice of pharmaceutical care. As you investigate or gain experience with different practice settings over your career, give some thought to how you can begin to implement some of the features of pharmaceutical care into a hospital practice. Although hospital practice, and especially clinical pharmacy, has always held itself to be dedicated to patient care, hospital pharmacists often find themselves thinking of the physician as their primary client rather than the patient. Taking the time to speak directly with patients can turn an already rewarding area of practice into a genuine patient care career.

Self Assessment: Patient Case Studies

Use the following patient case studies to answer these questions.

1. After reading just the one-paragraph summary of each case, what additional information do you want to collect? What will be the source of that information?

2. Based on the comprehensive case history provided, identify and prioritize any drug therapy problems you find. Is each drug therapy problem actual or potential?

3. Determine a goal for each drug therapy problem.

4. Identify at least two ways to resolve/prevent each drug therapy problem.

5. Choose the best option, justify your choice, and create a care plan. Your care plan should include monitoring and follow-up parameters.

6. Determine how you will implement your care plan.

7. Write a SOAP note to document your patient care activities.

Patient: Tommy Lohse

You are the clinical pharmacist on the pediatrics service at Memorial Hospital. Tommy, one of the children on your service, will be discharged home this afternoon (7/10/this year) after a 3 day admission. You have been asked to perform discharge counseling for Tommy and his mother. The physician's assistant's discharge note states that Tommy was admitted for treatment of osteomyelitis and he will be discharged on ceftazidime 1 g intravenously via peripherally inserted central catheter (PICC) line every 8 hours x 14 days. The hospital's home care pharmacy and nursing staff will prepare and administer his medication.

Tommy Lohse Case History

- **Chief Complaint:** Patient is experiencing pain in his right great toe. He has been diagnosed with osteomyelitis caused by Pseudomonas aeruginosa.

- **History of Present Illness:** Eight to 10 days prior to admission (approximately 6/28/this year) the patient punctured his foot through his running shoe while walking near a pond on his uncle's farm. Several days later, he complained of foot pain. He was originally seen by his pediatrician Dr. Ackley on 7/3/this year who placed him on amoxicillin/clavulanic acid 250/62.5 mg po q8h x 7 days and administered ceftriaxone 250 mg IM x 1. The patient's pain worsened and he was then given a second 250 mg dose of IM ceftriaxone by Dr. Ackley who referred the patient to an orthopedist, Dr. Bonnard, with a suspected diagnosis of osteomyelitis. Dr. Bonnard then performed an MRI which confirmed the diagnosis of osteomyelitis of the right great toe and he was admitted to the hospital on 7/7/this year.

  On 7/8/this year the patient underwent surgery where the infection was debrided and tissue was sent for culture and sensitivity. Culture was positive for Pseudomonas aeruginosa, sensitive to imipenem, meropenem, ceftazidime, cefipime, tobramycin, and ciprofloxacin. A PICC line was placed and he was started on ceftazidime 1 gram every 8 hours for 2 weeks by Dr. Bonnard's physician's assistant Cherie Nguyen. Patient will be discharged on 7/10/this year also on heparin flush, 10 unit/mL, 1-2 mL IV after each dose of ceftazidime.

- **Past Medical History:** uneventful

- **Medication History:** Patient's discharge medications include: IV ceftazidime 1 gram every 8 hours via PICC line for 2 weeks, heparin flush, 10 unit/mL, 1-2 mL IV after each dose of ceftazidime. Past medications include amoxicillin/clavulanic acid and ceftriaxone. He takes no routine medications while at home.

- **Family and Social History:** Patient is in school and has several older siblings.

- **Physical Examination and Objective Information:** Patient is a 7-year-old male, 127 cm tall weighing 26.3 kg. Labs taken on 7/7/this year include: total white cell count 13,400/mm^3 with 78% granulocytes and 6% bands; erythrocyte sedimentation rate 35mm/hr; random blood glucose 94 mg/dL; serum creatinine 0.5 mg/dL. Physical exam on 7/7/this year is relevant for a temperature of 37.7° C. Right great toe is erythematous and inflamed. Patient complains of moderate foot pain. On 7/10/this year, his total white blood cell count was 10,400/mm^3 with 64% granulocytes and 1% bands and his temperature was 36.9°C. He is still complaining of moderate foot pain.

Patient: Jerome Sandborne

You are the clinical pharmacist on the psychiatry service at Suburban General Hospital. Your duties include doing routine chart review and medication admission history on all patients admitted to your service. Your role is to determine if patient admissions are potentially drug-related and to identify any problems that may interfere with appropriate drug therapy during the patient's admission and after discharge. Today, you are interviewing Jerome, a 24-year-old male admitted yesterday (5/18/this year) for acute onset of mania.

Jerome Sandborne Case History
- **Chief Complaint:** "My wife thinks I have a problem and I need to be here."

- **History of Present Illness:** Patient was voluntarily admitted to the psychiatry inpatient service on 5/18/this year for recent onset of mania. He reports a 2 year history of bipolar affective disorder. He reports little or no sleep for the last 5 days, increased spending ($1000 on clothes and expensive gifts), and increased activity (mowing 13-14 of his neighbor's lawns in addition to his usual 8 hour workday). His wife reports that he believes members of her family are millionaires and that he tried to buy a second house up the street. Recently he has been preoccupied with religion.

- **Past Medical History:** NKDA. No chronic medical conditions or past surgeries. Two-year history of bipolar affective disorder. No past suicide attempts.

- **Outpatient Medication History:**
  Paroxetine 20 mg po qd.
  Lithium carbonate 300 mg po bid.
  Valproic Acid Delayed Release 500 mg po tid.

- **Medications on Admission:**
  Paroxetine 20 mg po qd.
  Lithium carbonate 300 mg po bid.
  Valproic Acid Delayed Release 500 mg po tid.
  Risperidone 2 mg po qhs, repeat x 1 prn.

- **Family History:** Older sister with schizophrenia.

- **Social History:** Positive for cannabis ("7-8 hitters/day" for unspecified period of time), last use 3 months ago, no history of other street drugs. Positive for tobacco. Minimal alcohol use. Married 3 years, employed as a warehouse worker. Has minimal health insurance and no prescription drug coverage.

- **Objective Info:** He presented with mania, grandiosity and religiosity, and a full, labile affect. He was alert and oriented x 3. He displayed pressured, tangential speech with overt paranoid and religious focus ("The vision God has given me is so big, I don't want anyone to miss it.") and flight-of-ideas.
  Axis I: Bipolar affective disorder with mania r/o current substance abuse.
  Axis II: Deferred.
  Axis III: None active.
  Axis IV: Mild problems with primary support and finances.
  Axis V: GAF = 35.

- **Physical Exam:**
  Vital signs: Temperature 37°C, Heart Rate 96bpm, Respiratory Rate 12 breaths/minute, BP 130/84.
  Laboratories: Serum lithium level below detectable limits, Serum valproate level below detectable limits, Na 132mEq/L, K 4.2mEq/L, Cl 102mEq/L, CO_2 24mEq/L, BUN 16 mg/dL, Creatinine 0.9 mg/dL, Glucose (random) 92 mg/dL, Thyroid function tests within normal limits, VDRL negative.

- **Review of Symptoms:** Lost 19 pounds in last 2 months; no pain.

- **Mental Status Exam:** Alert and oriented x 3, good grooming and hygiene.

  Affect: Labile, irritable and expansive.

  Speech: Pressured and tangential with loose associations, hyper-religious, paranoid, and grandiose.

  He denies hallucinations, suicidal and homicidal ideation.

  Insight poor.

  Judgment impaired.

References

1. Otto CN, McCloskey W. Hospitals in McCarthy RL, Schafermeyer KW (eds). *Introduction to Health Care Delivery: A Primer for Pharmacists.* 2nd Edition. Gaithersburg, MD: Aspen Publications; 2001:222-4.

Applying Clinical Skills in Long-Term-Care Settings

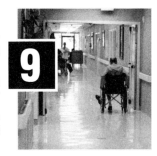

9

John P. Rovers

o many pharmacists, the phrase "long-term-care" probably means "nursing home." Although most long-term-care pharmacists (usually called consultant pharmacists) do serve nursing homes, these pharmacists practice in a wide variety of settings. Practice environments include both community-based and institutional locations. Some examples of long-term-care settings include nursing facilities (the preferred term for what are usually called nursing homes), skilled nursing facilities, adult day services, hospices, senior centers, correctional facilities, and home health care centers.[1]

In addition, the patient population served by consultant pharmacists is more diverse than most pharmacists imagine. Most patients cared for by consultant pharmacists are elderly, but other patient groups would include the chronically ill, patients undergoing rehabilitation for an acute illness, and the terminally ill.[2]

The diversity of care settings and patient populations notwithstanding, most consultant pharmacists provide clinical services to elderly residents of nursing facilities (NFs). Therefore, that is the focus of this chapter and the self assessments you will complete to test your pharmaceutical care skills.

Depending on where they work, pharmacists serving long-term-care facilities may provide only drug distribution services, only clinical services, or both. The practice of long-term-care pharmacy has evolved substantially over the last 30 years and most consultant pharmacists now find themselves working to meet a wide variety of complex federal mandates designed to protect the health and well-being of what is often a frail and vulnerable patient population.[2,3] Pharmacists caring for patients living in NFs are especially affected by such legislation. However, one positive result of these evolving regulations is that long-term-care pharmacy provides an exceptionally attractive opportunity to provide pharmaceutical care.

The patient population served by consultant pharmacists is more diverse than most pharmacists imagine.

Consultant pharmacists must realize that drug therapy in the elderly is not the same as drug therapy in other adults.

There is a bit of conceptual overlap between NF practice and inpatient pharmacy practice (see Chapter 8). In both cases, there is a strong tradition of pharmacists providing significant patient care. Also in both cases, pharmacists have easier access to both nurses and physicians than they do in the community setting. There is a comprehensive medical record for all patients in both practice environments as well, so collecting patient data is not overly difficult.

There are also some differences across these practice settings. Hospitalized inpatients may have 3- or 4-day stays, but long-term-care residents are there for weeks to years. As a result, consultant pharmacists can develop deeper relationships with their long-term-care patients and not have some of the time pressures inherent in providing pharmaceutical care to a hospital inpatient. Another point of difference may be the amount of objective data available to the pharmacist. Laboratory tests for most NF residents are performed only occasionally, not daily as they are for hospitalized patients. As a result, the pharmacist may have to make drug use decisions without knowing, for example, a resident's current renal or hepatic function.

It has been said that "any symptom in an elderly patient should be considered a drug side effect until proved otherwise."[4] Too often, health status changes in the elderly are simply considered to be the inevitable effects of aging. Sometimes, however, such changes are a result of poor drug use decision-making.

Consultant pharmacists must keep a number of factors in mind as they assess an aged patient's drug therapy. As people age, numerous physiological parameters that affect drug therapy change. Renal and hepatic function decline. Body weight and the ratio of fat to lean body mass change. Co-morbidities may result in a variety of drug–disease interactions and other medications can cause drug–drug interactions. Numerous drugs should be avoided when possible, and consultant pharmacists must be able to determine the safety of an existing medication and recommend alternatives if it is unsafe.[5] Simply put, a consultant pharmacist must realize that drug therapy in the elderly is not the same as drug therapy in other adults. Their patients are generally sicker and frailer. They may also take more medication and their cases are often more medically complex.

The most common clinical service consultant pharmacists provide to NF residents is the Drug Regimen Review (DRR).[3,6,7] This service is common in part because it is a federal requirement for NFs and in part because it is a quick and convenient way to begin providing patient care. The DRR has several goals. It should result in improved quality of care and better control of chronic illnesses. The resident's quality of life should improve and her functional status should be maintained or improved, and she should be able to avoid adverse drug reactions and additional health care costs.

Clark et al.[6] have provided a framework for DRR. When performing DRR, pharmacists should look for the following types of problems:

- Drug use without indication.

- Untreated indications.

- Improper drug selection.

- Subtherapeutic dosage.

- Overdosage.

- Adverse drug reactions.

- Drug interactions.

- Medication errors.

- Incomplete medication monitoring.

- High medication costs.

When performing DRR, pharmacists look for these problems by reviewing the patient's medication profile. Although it is not recommended, current guidelines for DRR state that a pharmacist is permitted to perform up to 100 DRR in any given day.[3] Pharmacists must ensure that they maintain a safe workload when performing DRR.

If this framework and profile review constitute the usual parameters of DRR, how closely does such a practice conform to the provision of pharmaceutical care? Recall that the practice of pharmaceutical care is the identification and prevention or resolution of drug therapy problems (DTPs).

The first seven problems listed in the framework for DRR above are essentially six of the seven DTPs described in Chapter 2 (see Table 2-1). The DTP taxonomy would categorize the seventh framework problem of drug interactions as a subset of either "dosage too high," "dosage too low," or "adverse effect."

The only DTP missing from the framework is noncompliance. If all a pharmacist's patients are residents of a facility where medications are administered by nursing staff, then this problem should never arise. As described above, however, not all patients are necessarily residents of such facilities, so this could be an important oversight in the framework, depending on the practice setting. The tenth framework problem of high medication costs, however, is described in the DTP taxonomy as a possible cause of noncompliance, so the framework does address the DTP of noncompliance, albeit incompletely.

Conversely, the new Medicare Part D program that provides prescription drug insurance for seniors is an excellent opportunity for pharmacists to discuss drug therapy with elderly patients. Although the discussion may initially focus on cost, pharmacists should use part of the conversation to screen the patient for any drug therapy problems, whether or not such problems may be related to prescription costs. Certainly, the framework's evaluation of medication cost-related problems can be considered to become an entry point for an assessment of possible DTPs.

The remaining items listed in the framework problems are medication errors and incomplete medication monitoring.

The pharmaceutical care process would also address incomplete medication monitoring, but differently. Suppose, for example, that a diabetic patient has never been evaluated for proteinuria. The framework identifies this as inherently a problem of incomplete monitoring. Using a pharmaceutical care approach, it remains an important matter, but would be considered to be an example of a poor-quality care plan in which the pharmacist did not adequately determine appropriate patient follow-up procedures. In other words, it is not a problem in and of itself, but rather evidence that the pharmacist did not provide optimal pharmaceutical care.

The last framework problem of medication errors is simply not addressed by the DTP taxonomy. Medication errors represent a problem with the medication use system. DTPs, on the other hand, represent problems that patients have. Although problems with medication systems are important and have a significant impact on patient care, they are conceptually outside the pharmaceutical care model which focuses exclusively on patients and ignores systems.

When the DRR framework and the DTP taxonomy are compared like this, it is apparent that the conceptual overlap between the two, although not complete, is substantial. The DRR framework is certainly congruent with the practice of pharmaceutical care.

There are differences, however, in how DRR and pharmaceutical care are performed. DRR can be performed without speaking with the patient. In contrast, pharmaceutical care practitioners develop a therapeutic relationship (see Chapter 3) with their patients, involving them in conversations that help them identify and solve problems in a patient-specific manner. When a pharmacist talks with a patient, it soon becomes clear that what may be a problem or a solution in one patient may not be a problem or a solution in another.

No doubt consultant pharmacists practicing DRR realize this as well. The difference is that a pharmaceutical care provider would talk to a patient as a matter of routine practice while a DRR provider would generally do so only if a profile review suggested there was a reason to. DRR providers also have to deal with the reality that many of their patients suffer from dementia or other conditions that make a meaningful conversation difficult or impossible. In such cases, the pharmacist should see if there are other members of the health care team or family members who can act as the patient's surrogate.

Ultimately, long-term-care pharmacy and pharmaceutical care are very similar models of practice. The problems that practitioners seek to find and fix are nearly identical. Given the large numbers of patients to whom consultant pharmacists provide care and the health status of many of them, it is not reasonable to expect consultants to discuss drug therapy with each patient. But when consultant pharmacists go beyond basic DRRs and speak with patients, understand their goals for their health and drug therapy, and individualize that therapy, then long-term-care pharmacy becomes synonymous with pharmaceutical care.

Ultimately, long-term-care pharmacy and pharmaceutical care are very similar models of practice.

Self Assessment: Patient Case Studies

Use the following patient case studies to answer these questions.

1. After reading just the one-paragraph summary of each case, what additional information do you want to collect? What will be the source of that information?

2. Based on the comprehensive case history provided, identify and prioritize any drug therapy problems you find. Is each drug therapy problem actual or potential?

3. Determine a goal for each drug therapy problem.

4. Identify at least two ways to resolve/prevent each drug therapy problem.

5. Choose the best option, justify your choice, and create a care plan. Your care plan should include monitoring and follow-up parameters.

6. Determine how you will implement your care plan.

7. Write a SOAP note to document your patient care activities.

Patient: Roberta Corrigan

You are a staff pharmacist at Mid-Town Drug and also serve as the consultant pharmacist for The Knightsbridge Home, which is a nursing facility. Roberta Corrigan was admitted two weeks ago on 10/17/this year. Today, (10/30/this year) you are performing an admission DRR and pharmaceutical care evaluation for Mrs. Corrigan. You have Mrs. Corrigan's demographic information, a medication profile, and medical problem list available at the pharmacy. Admission protocols at the home require a baseline laboratory panel to be drawn for each resident.

- **Demographics:**
  Date of birth 8/8/36
  Allergies and sensitivities: metformin (caused diarrhea), pioglitazone (caused edema), fosinopril (caused hyperkalemia). Height 5'1" Weight 53 kg.

- **Medical Problem List:**
  Type 2 diabetes mellitus.
  Diabetic nephropathy.
  Hypertension.
  Peripheral vascular disease.

Iron deficiency anemia.
Hyperlipidemia.
Osteoporosis.

- **Current Medications:**
  Simvastatin 40 mg qd.
  Hydrochlorothiazide 25 mg qd.
  Glyburide 10 mg bid.
  Oyster calcium 500 mg bid.
  Alendronate 70 mg q Monday.
  Amlodipine 10 mg qd.
  Nabumetone 500 mg bid.
  Cyanocobalamin 1000 mcg IM q monthly.
  Ferrous sulfate 325 mg qd.
  Loratidine 10 mg qd.
  Influenza vaccine on admission.

Roberta Corrigan Case History
- **Vital Signs:** BP 138/80; HR 100, RR 12, T 98.8.

- **Lipids:** Total cholesterol 190 mg/dL, Triglycerides 121 mg/dL, HDL 48 mg/dL, LDL 66 mg/dL.

- **Chemistries:** Na 140mEq/L, K 4.8mEq/L, Cl 110mEq/L, CO_2 22 mEq/L, BUN 21mg/dL, Cr 1.4mg/dL (calculated creatinine clearance 31mL/min), Random glucose 138mg/dL, Hemoglobin A1c 7.3%, ALT 17U/L, AST 24U/L, Total bilirubin 0.6 mg/dL, Alkaline Phosphatase 44U/L, Uric Acid 6.4 mg/dL, Urinary protein 16 mg/dL, Ca 8.8 mg/dL, Mg 2.0mEq/L, Phosphorus 3.2 mg/dL, Albumin 4.4g/L.

- **Hematologies:** Hemoglobin 10.2g/L, Hematocrit 30.8%, WBC 5600/mm³, 70% Neutrophils, 26% Lymphocytes, Platelets 168,000/mm³, Serum Iron 48mcg/dL, Total Iron Binding Capacity 460mcg/dL, Mean Corpuscular Volume 90fL.

Patient: Jacob Hensler

On 9/22/this year, you receive a fax from Juno House, the nursing facility at which you are the consultant pharmacist. The fax is a copy of the physician's orders for that day for one of the residents, Jacob Hensler, and it reads "d/c atorvastatin." You make a note to yourself to evaluate the situation during your next DRR session for Juno House which is scheduled for next week. In previous DRRs you determined that Mr. Hensler's current drug therapy has been both safe and effective and that he is generally satisfied with it. Meanwhile, you quickly review Mr. Hensler's current profile and note the following:

Medication	Directions	Indication
Amiodarone100 mg	1 tab QD	Arrhythmia
Glimepiride 2 mg	1 tab QD	Type 2 diabetes
Atorvastatin 20 mg	1 tab QD	Hyperlipidemia
Furosemide 40 mg	1 tab QD	CHF
Fluoxetine 20 mg	1 cap QD	Depression
ASA/Dipyridamole 25/200	1 cap BID	TIA prophylaxis
Losartan 50 mg	1 tab QD	CHF, Type 2 diabetes
Acetaminophen 500 mg	2 tabs prn	Pain
Diazepam 2.5 mg	1 tab QD and QHS PRN	Anxiety/insomnia
Becomethasone 40 mcg MDI	2 puffs BID	COPD

Allergies: NKDA

Jacob Hensler Case History
• **Past Medical History:** Edema, Arrythmia, Type 2 Diabetes, Congestive Heart Failure, Depression, Transient Ischemic Attacks, Insomnia, Chronic Obstructive Pulmonary Disease.

• **Allergies:** NKA.

• **Family History/Social History:** N/A.

• **Objective Information:**
Lipid profile 6/20/this year: Total cholesterol 188 mg/dL, LDL 88 mg/dL, HDL 44 mg/dL, TG 133 mg/dL.
Blood pressure: 9/21/this year 124/74, 9/14/this year 126/70, 9/7/this year 118/50.
Liver function tests from 9/21/this year: ALT 288U/L, AST 302U/L, Alkaline Phosphatase 249U/L,
Total bilirubin 0.7 mg/dL, Prothrombin time 12 seconds.
Thyroid function tests from 5/1/this year: Free T_4 1.2ng/dL, TSH 3.3mIU/mL.
Blood glucose from 9/21 (random) 104 mg/dL.
Electrolytes from 9/21/this year: Na 142mEq/L, K 3.3mEq/L, Cl 98mEq/L, CO_2 26mEq/L.
BUN and Creatinine from 9/21/this year: 22 mg/dL and 0.8 mg/dL respectively.

References

1. Knight-Klimas TC, Stefanacci RG. Pharmacist Involvement in Long Term Care for Seniors in *Pharmacy and the US Health Care System,* 3rd Edition. Smith MI, Wertheimer AI, Fincham JE, eds. Binghampton, NY: Pharmaceutical Products Press; 2005:193-226.

2. Plake KS, Dole EJ. Long Term Care in *Introduction to Health Care Delivery: A Primer for Pharmacists,* 2nd Edition. McCarthy RL, Schafermeyer KW, eds. Gaithersburg, MD: Aspen Publishers; 2001:255-76.

3. Clark TR, Gruber J, Sey M. Revisiting Drug Regimen Review Part 1: The Early History and Evolution of DRR. *Consult Pharm.* 2003;18:215-20.

4. Gurwitz J, Monane M, Monane S, et al. Polypharmacy in *Quality Care in the Nursing Home.* Morris JN, Lipsitz LA, Murphy K, et al., eds. St. Louis, MO: Mosby Year Book; 1997:13-25.

5. Beers MH. Explicit Criteria for Determining Potentially Inappropriate Medication Use by the Elderly: An Update. *Arch Intern Med.* 1997;157:1531-6.

6. Clark TR, Gruber J, Sey M. Revisiting Drug Regimen Review Part 2: Art or Science? *Consult Pharm.* 2003;18:506-13.

7. Clark TR, Gruber J, Sey M. Revisiting Drug Regimen Review Part 3: A Systematic Approach to Drug Regimen Review. *Consult Pharm.* 2003;18:657-66.

Notes

Applying Clinical Skills in Clinics or Ambulatory Settings

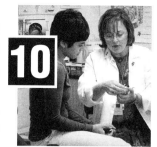

Jay D. Currie and CoraLynn B. Trewet

The information in this chapter and the accompanying cases test your patient care skills in clinics or ambulatory practice settings. In these settings the pharmacist may be the primary care provider, or she may work closely with another provider. Currently only a small percentage of pharmacists are working in clinics or ambulatory practices, but that is changing. An increased focus on quality and safety in medication use, along with other Medication Therapy Management Service (MTMS) strategies, may cause the number to increase.

Pharmacists practicing in clinics and ambulatory settings (which may include free-standing centers and clinics associated with health systems) provide care in an environment that is most often devoid of any product distribution. These pharmacists may be practicing independently as the primary provider for the clinic. Or they may be one of many providers working together in a multispecialty practice. Clinical settings may focus on a set of disease states, like anticoagulation or warfarin management, hypertension, hyperlipidemia, asthma, or diabetes mellitus. Or they may focus on issues of particular concern to their patients, including geriatrics, complex medication management, smoking cessation, and pain management.

While this nontraditional form of pharmacy practice has existed for several years, collaborative practice agreements and payment for pharmacist services have increased pharmacist involvement in the primary care setting. These agreements have also created opportunities for community pharmacies to establish ambulatory care services.

These practice settings differ from others in the nature of the interaction between the pharmacist and other care providers,

Pharmacists practicing in clinics and ambulatory settings (which may include free-standing centers and clinics associated with health systems) provide care in an environment that is most often devoid of any product distribution.

and also in the availability of data. In ambulatory care settings, pharmacists and other providers often work side-by-side throughout the day. Unlike the community pharmacy where communication is facilitated through telephone calls and faxes, this setting allows for seamless communication.

In this fast-paced environment, however, the time available for providers to interact may be limited. Even if this is the case, the setting does allow for an easier flow of information than if the pharmacist is communicating from outside the organization.

Access to patient information in these settings is often the same or nearly equivalent to what a physician would have in an office setting. If pharmacists are part of a multispecialty group, they are likely using the same records as the other providers. Whether in a paper charting system or an electronic medical record (EMR), provider notes from previous patient encounters, including diagnoses and care plans, are likely available. Chronologically recorded vital signs, laboratory results, and health maintenance information is probably also accessible. Having access to correspondence with consultants and other providers outside the practice, in addition to hospitalization histories, physicals, and discharge summaries, allows the pharmacist to obtain more complete information about the patient. In a pharmacist-only staffed clinic, the quality of the patient record may depend on the documentation skills of the pharmacist providers.

Information from patients or their caregivers may also be more easily obtained in this setting. A pharmacist using a more complete patient record can spend more time getting the specific information she needs. She can simply fill in the gaps not included in the patient record rather than concentrating on collecting the entire database. Interacting with the patient in a private room in a professional setting may allow for an easier exchange of information.

Room availability, clinic space, patient scheduling patterns, and the pace of care delivered in the clinic are all variables that affect the pharmacist–patient encounter. A productive, positive experience with a patient will usually result in more useful data.

Having access to more information is both a blessing and a curse. Sometimes the extra information can make working with the patient more complex and confusing, making it difficult for the pharmacist to determine the true clinical picture of the patient. Sorting additional information can also consume considerable time and distract the pharmacist from more pressing issues. The pharmacist must determine what information is needed to provide care to the patient and what information does not need to be considered in the current circumstances. Extraneous information such as irrelevant laboratory tests or medical history that isn't currently an issue for the patient can be as perplexing as a lack of information.

The pharmacist's ability to collect specimens and perform laboratory testing would depend on the clinical setting, but would likely be more extensive than in community pharmacy practice. Having ready access to laboratory or other diagnostic testing requires the pharmacist to know when to utilize the testing, how to interpret the results, and ultimately how to provide appropriate care from those results.

Learning what information you need, where you can find it, and how to sort out relevant from irrelevant data are all important factors in providing care to patients in any setting. In working through the cases in this chapter, think about what information you will gather from charts and what information you will need to collect from patients.

Room availability, clinic space, patient scheduling patterns, and the pace of care delivered in the clinic are all variables that will affect the pharmacist–patient encounter.

Self Assessment: Patient Case Studies

Use the following patient case studies to answer these questions.

1. After reading just the one-paragraph summary of each case, what additional information do you want to collect? What will be the source of that information?

2. Based on the comprehensive case history provided, identify and prioritize any drug therapy problems you find. Is each drug therapy problem actual or potential?

3. Determine a goal for each drug therapy problem.

4. Identify at least two ways to resolve/prevent each drug therapy problem.

5. Choose the best option, justify your choice, and create a care plan. Your care plan should include monitoring and follow-up parameters.

6. Determine how you will implement your care plan.

7. Write a SOAP note to document your patient care activities.

Patient: Fred Willert

As the clinical pharmacist working at your health system's Diabetes Care Center, you see patients at routine interval visits for medication assessment and adjustment between those with the endocrinologist and the diabetes team. Fred Willert, your second patient today (10/23/this year) presented for his first follow-up visit after completing the initial educational program and plan implementation. You look at the patient chart and see the medical assistant has recorded the following:

- 10/23/this year: BP 132/80, Pulse 78, Wt. 236 lbs, Ht. 5'7", Fasting BG 138.

- **Chief Complaint:** Trouble adjusting to the small portion sizes/ new meal plan, and difficulty taking his meds.

Fred Willert Case History
- **Chief Complaint:** Patient presented to the Diabetes Center on 10/23/this year for his initial follow-up visit. He reports having trouble adjusting to the small portion sizes of the new meal plan and also is having trouble taking his diabetic medication regularly.

- **History of Present Illness:** Patient is a 49-year-old white male diagnosed with Type 2 diabetes mellitus 9/12/this year by his primary care physician, when he was found to have a random blood glucose of 272 mg/dL and blood pressure of 158/94 mmHg. He had an initial assessment at the Diabetes Center on 9/22/ this year where he was given classes teaching him about diabetes mellitus, blood glucose monitoring, diet, and meal planning. At the 9/22 visit he was also diagnosed with hypertension as his blood pressure remained elevated at 152/82 mmHg. He was started on an ACEI plus diuretic per JNC7 hypertension guidelines.

  Patient comes to his appointment today stating that he often gets up too late in the morning to eat breakfast so he doesn't take his metformin, but takes his lisinopril/hydrochlorothiazide. He then does not take the medication to work with him so he does not take it at lunch either. If he does remember to take it, it is usually with dinner, which is very late at times.

  From talking with the patient and looking at his diabetes record/ blood glucose daily log, it's clear he has only taken about 6 doses of metformin since starting it 9/22/this year. He also states that the meal plan is somewhat challenging, especially with eating the smaller portions. He wonders if he can add the carbs that he does not use for snacks during the day to dinner at night. He is adjusting to the new lifestyle and diagnosis and is willing to keep trying. He is unable to take another foods class offered by the Center because of cost. He is not willing to try and quit smoking at this time due to overwhelming adjustment to diagnosis.

- **Past Medication History:**
  Type 2 diabetes mellitus x 1.5 months.
  HTN x 1 month.

- **Social History:** Lives at home alone. He is rushed in the morning hours getting ready for work because he likes to get there early to socialize. He admits to smoking a little over a pack of cigarettes a day and estimates that he has about 10 alcoholic beverages per week.

- **Family History:** Mother diagnosed with DM at 55 y.o. and father had a heart attack at 62 y.o.

- **Medication List:**
  Metformin 500 mg po BID with meals (see above).
  Lisinopril/Hydrochlorothiazide 20/12.5 mg po QDay (takes daily in am).
  MVI QDay (takes daily in am).
  Aspirin 81 mg QDay (takes daily, heard it was good for him).

- **Vital Signs:** Today BP 132/80, Wt. 236 lbs, Ht. 5'7",
  BMI 36.9, BG 138.
  9/24/this year   Microalbuminuria 8.5.
  9/22/this year   BP 152/82.
  9/12/this year   HbA1c 8.5, Random BG 232, BP 158/94.
  9/9/this year   TC 176, HDL 34, LDL 93, TG 245.

Patient: Allison Chance

As the clinical pharmacist working at an Anticoagulation Clinic, you see patients on warfarin therapy at weekly to monthly intervals to adjust their dose per their International Normalized Ratio (INR). Allison Chance, a patient you have had since you started at the clinic, presents today (10/23/this year), one month after her last visit. You look at the patient chart and see the medical assistant has recorded the following:

- 10/23/this year   BP 120/78, Pulse 66 Irregular, Wt. 178 lbs, Ht. 5'8", INR 1.7.

- **Chief Complaint:** No complaints. She just went on a diet in preparation for a trip to the Caribbean.

Allison Chance Case History
- **Chief Complaint:** Patient presented to the Anticoagulation Clinic on 10/23/this year for scheduled follow-up visit. She does not have any complaints but mentions she has recently gone on a diet.

- **History of Present Illness:** Allison is a 40-year-old white female diagnosed with atrial fibrillation during an episode of chest pain at the emergency room three years ago. At that time she was started on appropriate rate control and anticoagulation therapy. For three years her INR has been within the goal range of 2.0-3.0 most of the time, however is low today at 1.7. While talking to this patient you learn she started a diet two weeks ago. She states that she eats lots of salads and is taking an herbal medication to help lose weight. She wants to continue the dietary changes as she thinks it is helping her control her calorie intake.

- **Past Medication History:**
  Atrial fibrillation x 3 years.
  Hypertension x 4 years.

- **Social History:** Married with two children. She does not smoke. She usually has a glass of red wine with dinner because she heard it was good for her heart.

- Family History: Both parents are alive and healthy. Brother had heart attack one year ago (age of 49).

- Medication List:
  Warfarin 5 mg daily (takes daily at bedtime).
  Diltiazem 240 mg bid (takes daily in am and bedtime).
  Calcium 600 mg bid (takes daily in am and bedtime).
  Herbal diet medication, unsure of ingredients (takes daily in am).

- Vital Signs:
  Today BP 120/78, Pulse 66 Irregular, Wt. 178 lbs, Ht. 5'8", INR 1.7.
  9/24/this year INR 2.6.
  8/25/this year INR 2.5.
  7/26/this year INR 2.6.

Appendix A

American Pharmaceutical Association
Principles of Practice for Pharmaceutical Care

Preamble

Pharmaceutical care is a patient-centered, outcomes oriented pharmacy practice that requires the pharmacist to work in concert with the patient and the patient's other healthcare providers to promote health, to prevent disease, and to assess, monitor, initiate, and modify medication use to assure that drug therapy[1] regimens are safe and effective. The goal of pharmaceutical care is to optimize the patient's health-related quality of life, and achieve positive clinical outcomes, within realistic economic expenditures. To achieve this goal, the following must be accomplished:

A. A professional relationship must be established and maintained.

Interaction between the pharmacist and the patient must occur to assure that a relationship based upon caring, trust, open communication, cooperation, and mutual decision making is established and maintained. In this relationship, the pharmacist holds the patient's welfare paramount, maintains an appropriate attitude of caring for the patient's welfare, and uses all his/her professional knowledge and skills on the patient's behalf. In exchange, the patient agrees to supply personal information and preferences, and participate in the therapeutic plan. The pharmacist develops mechanisms to assure the patient has access to pharmaceutical care at all times.

B. Patient-specific medical information must be collected, organized, recorded, and maintained.

Pharmacists must collect and/or generate subjective and objective information regarding the patient's general health and activity status, past medical history, medication history, social history, diet and exercise history, history of present illness, and economic situation (financial and insured status). Sources of information may include, but are not limited to, the patient, medical charts and reports, pharmacist-conducted health/physical assessment, the patient's family or caregiver, insurer, and other healthcare providers including physicians, nurses, mid-level practitioners and other pharmacists. Since this information will form the basis for deci-

---

1. Although "drug therapy" typically refers to intended, beneficial effects of pharmacologic drugs, in this document, "drug therapy" refers to the intended, beneficial use of drugs—whether diagnostic or therapeutic—and thus includes diagnostic radiopharmaceuticals, X-ray contrast media, etc. in addition to pharmacologic drugs. Similarly, "drug therapy plan" includes the outcomes-oriented plan for diagnostic drug use in addition to pharmacologic drug use.

sions regarding the development and subsequent modification of the drug therapy plan, it must be timely, accurate, and complete, and it must be organized and recorded to assure that it is readily retrievable and updated as necessary and appropriate. Patient information must be maintained in a confidential manner.

C. Patient-specific medical information must be evaluated and a drug therapy plan developed mutually with the patient.

Based upon a thorough understanding of the patient and his/her condition or disease and its treatment, the pharmacist must, with the patient and with the patient's other healthcare providers as necessary, develop an outcomes-oriented drug therapy plan. The plan may have various components which address each of the patient's diseases or conditions. In designing the plan, the pharmacist must carefully consider the psychosocial aspects of the disease as well as the potential relationship between the cost and/or complexity of therapy and patient adherence. As one of the patient's advocates, the pharmacist assures the coordination of drug therapy with the patient's other healthcare providers and the patient. In addition, the patient must be apprised of (1) various pros and cons (i.e., cost, side effects, different monitoring aspects, etc.) of the options relative to drug therapy and (2) instances where one option may be more beneficial based on the pharmacist's professional judgment. The essential elements of the plan, including the patient's responsibilities, must be carefully and completely explained to the patient. Information should be provided to the patient at a level the patient will understand. The drug therapy plan must be documented in the patient's pharmacy record and communicated to the patient's other healthcare providers as necessary.

D.The pharmacist assures that the patient has all supplies, information, and knowledge necessary to carry out the drug therapy plan.

The pharmacist providing pharmaceutical care must assume ultimate responsibility for assuring that his/her patient has been able to obtain, and is appropriately using, any drugs and related products or equipment called for in the drug therapy plan. The pharmacist must also assure that the patient has a thorough understanding of the disease and the therapy/medications prescribed in the plan.

E. The pharmacist reviews, monitors, and modifies the therapeutic plan as necessary and appropriate, in concert with the patient and healthcare team.

The pharmacist is responsible for monitoring the patient's progress in achieving the specific outcomes according to strategy developed in the drug therapy plan. The pharmacist coordinates changes in the plan with the patient and the patient's other healthcare providers as necessary and appropriate in order to maintain or enhance the safety and/or effectiveness of drug therapy and to help minimize overall healthcare costs. Patient progress is accurately documented in the pharmacy record and communicated to the patient and to the patient's other healthcare providers as appropriate. The pharmacist shares information with other healthcare providers as the setting for care changes, thus helping assure continuity of care as the patient moves between the community setting, the institutional setting, and the long-term-care setting.

Practice Principles

1. Data Collection

1.1 The pharmacist conducts an initial interview with the patient for the purposes of establishing a professional working relationship and initiating the patient's pharmacy record. In some situations (e.g., pediatrics, geriatrics, critical care, language barriers) the opportunity to develop a professional relationship with and collect information directly from the patient may not exist. Under these circumstances, the pharmacist should work directly with the patient's parent, guardian, and/or principal caregiver.

1.2 The interview is organized, professional, and meets the patient's need for confidentiality and privacy. Adequate time is devoted to assure that questions and answers can be fully developed without either party feeling uncomfortable or hurried. The interview is used to systematically collect patient-specific subjective information and to initiate a pharmacy record which includes information and data regarding the patient's general health and activity status, past medical history, medication history, social history (including economic situation), family history, and history of present illness. The record should also include information regarding the patient's thoughts or feelings and perceptions of his/her condition or disease.

1.3 The pharmacist uses health/physical assessment techniques (blood-pressure monitoring, etc.) appropriately and as necessary to acquire necessary patient-specific objective information.

1.4 The pharmacist uses appropriate secondary sources to supplement the information obtained through the initial patient interview and health/physical assessment. Sources may include, but are not limited to, the patient's medical record or medical reports, the patient's family, and the patient's other healthcare providers.

1.5 The pharmacist creates a pharmacy record for the patient and accurately records the information collected. The pharmacist assures that the patient's record is appropriately organized, kept current, and accurately reflects all pharmacist–patient encounters. The confidentiality of the information in the record is carefully guarded and appropriate systems are in place to assure security. Patient-identifiable information contained in the record is provided to others only upon the authorization of the patient or as required by law.

2. Information Evaluation

2.1 The pharmacist evaluates the subjective and objective information collected from the patient and other sources then forms conclusions regarding: (1) opportunities to improve and/or assure the safety, effectiveness, and/or economy of current or planned drug therapy; (2) opportunities to minimize current or potential future drug or health-related problems; and (3) the timing of any necessary future pharmacist consultation.

2.2 The pharmacist records the conclusions of the evaluation in the medical and/or pharmacy record.

2.3 The pharmacist discusses the conclusions with the patient, as necessary and appropriate, and assures an appropriate understanding of the nature of the condition or illness and what might be expected with respect to its management.

3. Formulating a Plan

3.1 The pharmacist, in concert with other healthcare providers, identifies, evaluates, and then chooses the most appropriate action(s) to: (1) improve and/or assure the safety, effectiveness, and/or cost-effectiveness of current or planned drug therapy; and/or (2) minimize current or potential future health-related problems.

3.2 The pharmacist formulates plans to effect the desired outcome. The plans may include, but are not limited to, work with the patient as well as with other health providers to develop a patient-specific drug therapy protocol or to modify prescribed drug therapy, develop and/or implement drug therapy monitoring mechanisms, recommend nutritional or dietary modifications, add nonprescription medications or nondrug treatments, refer the patient to an appropriate source of care, or institute an existing drug therapy protocol.

3.3 For each problem identified, the pharmacist actively considers the patient's needs and determines the desirable and mutually agreed upon outcome and incorporates these into the plan. The plan may include specific disease state and drug therapy endpoints and monitoring endpoints.

3.4 The pharmacist reviews the plan and desirable outcomes with the patient and with the patient's other healthcare provider(s) as appropriate.

3.5 The pharmacist documents the plan and desirable outcomes in the patient's medical and/or pharmacy record.

4. Implementing the Plan

4.1 The pharmacist and the patient take the steps necessary to implement the plan. These steps may include, but are not limited to, contacting other health providers to clarify or modify prescriptions, initiating drug therapy, educating the patient and/or caregiver(s), coordinating the acquisition of medications and/or related supplies, which might include helping the patient overcome financial barriers or lifestyle barriers that might otherwise interfere with the therapy plan, or coordinating appointments with other healthcare providers to whom the patient is being referred.

4.2 The pharmacist works with the patient to maximize patient understanding and involvement in the therapy plan, assures that arrangements for drug therapy monitoring (e.g., laboratory evaluation, blood pressure monitoring, home blood glucose testing, etc.) are made and understood by the patient, and that the patient receives and knows how to properly use all necessary medications and related equipment. Explanations are tailored to the patient's level of comprehension and teaching and adherence aids are employed as indicated.

4.3 The pharmacist assures that appropriate mechanisms are in place to ensure that the proper medications, equipment, and supplies are received by the patient in a timely fashion.

4.4 The pharmacist documents in the medical and/or pharmacy record the steps taken to implement the plan including the appropriate baseline monitoring parameters, and any barriers which will need to be overcome.

4.5 The pharmacist communicates the elements of the plan to the patient and/or the patient's other healthcare provider(s). The pharmacist shares information with other healthcare providers as the setting for care changes, in order to help maintain continuity of care as the patient moves between the ambulatory, inpatient, or long-term-care environment.

5. Monitoring and Modifying the Plan/Assuring Positive Outcomes

5.1 The pharmacist regularly reviews subjective and objective monitoring parameters in order to determine if satisfactory progress is being made toward achieving desired outcomes as outlined in the drug therapy plan.

5.2 The pharmacist and patient determine if the original plan should continue to be followed or if modifications are needed. If changes are necessary, the pharmacist works with the patient/caregiver and his/her other healthcare providers to modify and implement the revised plan as described in "Formulating a Plan" and "Implementing the Plan" above.

5.3 The pharmacist reviews ongoing progress in achieving desired outcomes with the patient and provides a report to the patient's other healthcare providers as appropriate. As progress towards outcomes is achieved, the pharmacist should provide positive reinforcement.

5.4 A mechanism is established for follow-up with patients. The pharmacist uses appropriate professional judgment in determining the need to notify the patient's other healthcare providers of the patient's level of adherence with the plan.

5.5 The pharmacist updates the patient's medical and/or pharmacy record with information concerning patient progress, noting the subjective and objective information which has been considered, his/her assessment of the patient's current progress, the patient's assessment of his/her current progress, and any modifications that are being made to the plan. Communications with other healthcare providers should also be noted.

Appendix

Pharmaceutical care is a process of drug therapy management that requires a change in the orientation of traditional professional attitudes and re-engineering of the traditional pharmacy environment. Certain elements of structure must be in place to provide quality pharmaceutical care. Some of these elements are: (1) knowledge, skill, and function of personnel, (2) systems for data collection, documentation, and transfer of information, (3) efficient work flow processes, (4) references, resources, and equipment, (5) communication skills, and (6) commitment to quality improvement and assessment procedures.

Knowledge, skill, and function of personnel

The implementation of pharmaceutical care is supported by knowledge and skills in the area of patient assessment, clinical information, communication, adult teaching and learning principles, and psychosocial aspects of care. To use these skills, responsibilities must be reassessed, and assigned to appropriate personnel, including pharmacists, technicians, automation, and technology. A mechanism of certifying and credentialling will support the implementation of pharmaceutical care.

Systems for data collection and documentation

The implementation of pharmaceutical care is supported by data collection and documentation systems that accommodate patient care communications (e.g., patient contact notes, medical/medication history), interprofessional communications (e.g., physician communication, pharmacist to pharmacist communication), quality assurance (e.g., patient outcomes assessment, patient care protocols), and research (e.g., data for pharmacoepidemiology, etc.). Documentation systems are vital for reimbursement considerations.

Efficient work flow processes

The implementation of pharmaceutical care is supported by incorporating patient care into the activities of the pharmacist and other personnel.

References, resources, and equipment

The implementation of pharmaceutical care is supported by tools which facilitate patient care, including equipment to assess medication therapy adherence and effectiveness, clinical resource materials, and patient education materials. Tools may include computer software support, drug utilization evaluation (DUE) programs, disease management protocols, etc.

Communication skills

The implementation of pharmaceutical care is supported by patient-centered communication. Within this communication, the patient plays a key role in the overall management of the therapy plan.

Quality assessment/improvement programs

The implementation and practice of pharmaceutical care is supported and improved by measuring, assessing, and improving pharmaceutical care activities utilizing the conceptual framework of continuous quality improvement.

Note:

This document will not cover each and every situation; that was not the intent of the Advisory Committee. This is a dynamic document and is intended to be revised as the profession adapts to its new role. It is hoped that pharmacists will use these principles, adapting them to their own situation and environments, to establish and implement pharmaceutical care.

Prepared by the APhA Pharmaceutical Care Guidelines Advisory Committee; approved by the APhA Board of Trustees, August 1995. © 1996 by the American Pharmaceutical Association. All rights reserved.

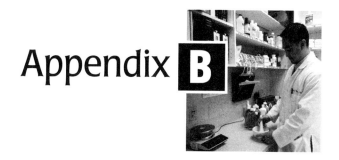

Appendix B

American Society of Health-System Pharmacists Statement on Pharmaceutical Care

The purpose of this statement is to assist pharmacists in understanding pharmaceutical care. Such understanding must precede efforts to implement pharmaceutical care, which ASHP believes merit the highest priority in all practice settings.

Possibly the earliest published use of the term pharmaceutical care was by Brodie in the context of thoughts about drug use control and medication-related services.[1,2] It is a term that has been widely used and a concept about which much has been written and discussed in the pharmacy profession, especially since the publication of a paper by Hepler and Strand in 1990.[3,5] ASHP has formally endorsed the concept.[6] With varying terminology and nuances, the concept has also been acknowledged by other national pharmacy organizations.[7,8] Implementation of pharmaceutical care was the focus of a major ASHP conference in March 1993.

Many pharmacists have expressed enthusiasm for the concept of pharmaceutical care, but there has been substantial inconsistency in its description. Some have characterized it as merely a new name for clinical pharmacy; others have described it as anything that pharmacists do that may lead to beneficial results for patients.

ASHP believes that pharmaceutical care is an important new concept that represents growth in the profession beyond clinical pharmacy as often practiced and beyond other activities of pharmacists, including medication preparation and dispensing. All of these professional activities are important, however, and ASHP continues to be a strong proponent of the necessity for pharmacists' involvement in them. In practice, these activities should be integrated with and culminate in pharmaceutical care provided by individual pharmacists to individual patients.

In 1992, ASHP's members urged the development of an officially recognized ASHP definition of pharmaceutical care.[9] This statement provides a definition and elucidates some of the elements and implications of that definition. The definition that follows is an adaptation of a definition developed by Hepler and Strand.[3]

Definition

The mission of the pharmacist is to provide pharmaceutical care. Pharmaceutical care is the direct, responsible provision of medication-related care for the purpose of achieving definite outcomes that improve a patient's quality of life.

Principal Elements

The principal elements of pharmaceutical care are that it is medication related; it is care that is directly provided to the patient; it is provided to produce definite outcomes; these outcomes are intended to improve the patient's quality of life; and the provider accepts personal responsibility for the outcomes.

Medication Related

Pharmaceutical care involves not only medication therapy (the actual provision of medication) but also decisions about medication use for individual patients. As appropriate, this includes decisions not to use medication therapy as well as judgments about medication selection, dosages, routes and methods of administration, medication therapy monitoring, and the provision of medication-related information and counseling to individual patients.

Care

Central to the concept of care is caring, a personal concern for the well-being of another person. Overall patient care consists of integrated domains of care including (among others) medical care, nursing care, and pharmaceutical care. Health professionals in each of these disciplines possess unique expertise and must cooperate in the patient's overall care. At times, they share in the execution of the various types of care (including pharmaceutical care). To pharmaceutical care, however, the pharmacist contributes unique knowledge and skills to ensure optimal outcomes from the use of medications.

At the heart of any type of patient care, there exists a one-to-one relationship between a caregiver and a patient. In pharmaceutical care, the irreducible "unit" of care is one pharmacist in a direct professional relationship with one patient. In this relationship, the pharmacist provides care directly to the patient and for the benefit of the patient.

The health and well-being of the patient are paramount. The pharmacist makes a direct, personal, caring commitment to the individual patient and acts in the patient's best interest. The pharmacist cooperates directly with other professionals and the patient in designing, implementing, and monitoring a therapeutic plan intended to produce definite therapeutic outcomes that improve the patient's quality of life.

Outcomes

It is the goal of pharmaceutical care to improve an individual patient's quality of life through achievement of definite (predefined), medication-related therapeutic outcomes. The outcomes sought are:

1. Cure of a patient's disease.

2. Elimination or reduction of a patient's symptomatology.

3. Arresting or slowing of a disease process.

4. Preventing a disease or symptomatology.

This, in turn, involves three major functions: (1) identifying potential and actual medication-related problems, (2) resolving actual medication-related problems, and (3) preventing potential medication-related problems. A medication-related problem is an event or circumstance involving medication therapy that actually or potentially interferes with an optimum outcome for a specific patient. There are at least the following categories of medication-related problems:[3]

- **Untreated indications.** The patient has a medical problem that requires medication therapy (an indication for medication use) but is not receiving a medication for that indication.

- **Improper drug selection.** The patient has a medication indication but is taking the wrong medication.

- **Subtherapeutic dosage.** The patient has a medical problem that is being treated with too little of the correct medication.

- **Failure to receive medication.** The patient has a medical problem that is the result of not receiving a medication (e.g., for pharmaceutical, psychological, sociological, or economic reasons).

- **Overdosage.** The patient has a medical problem that is being treated with too much of the correct medication (toxicity).

- **Adverse drug reactions.** The patient has a medical problem that is the result of an adverse drug reaction or adverse effect.

- **Drug interactions.** The patient has a medical problem that is the result of a drug–drug, drug–food, or drug–laboratory test interaction.

- **Medication use without indication.** The patient is taking a medication for no medically valid indication.

Patients may possess characteristics that interfere with the achievement of desired therapeutic outcomes. Patients may be noncompliant with prescribed medication use regimens, or there may be unpredictable variation in patients' biological responses. Thus, in an imperfect world, intended outcomes from medication-related therapy are not always achievable.

Patients bear a responsibility to help achieve the desired outcomes by engaging in behaviors that will contribute to—and not interfere with—the achievement of desired outcomes. Pharmacists and other health professionals have an obligation to educate patients about behaviors that will contribute to achieving desired outcomes.

Quality of Life

Some tools exist now for assessing a patient's quality of life. These tools are still evolving, and pharmacists should maintain familiarity with the literature on this subject.[10,11] A complete assessment of a patient's quality of life should include both objective and subjective (e.g., the patient's own) assessments. Patients should be involved, in an informed way, in establishing quality-of-life goals for their therapies.

Responsibility

The fundamental relationship in any type of patient care is a mutually beneficial exchange in which the patient grants authority to the provider and the provider gives competence and commitment to the patient (accepts responsibility).[3] Responsibility involves both moral trustworthiness and accountability.

In pharmaceutical care, the direct relationship between an individual pharmacist and an individual patient is that of a professional covenant in which the patient's safety and well-being are entrusted to the pharmacist, who commits to honoring that trust through competent professional actions that are in the patient's best interest. As an accountable member of the healthcare team, the pharmacist must document the care provided.[4,7,12,13] The pharmacist is personally accountable for patient outcomes (the quality of care) that ensue from the pharmacist's actions and decisions.[1]

Implications

The idea that pharmacists should commit themselves to the achievement of definite outcomes for individual patients is an especially important element in the concept of pharmaceutical care. The expectation that pharmacists personally accept responsibility for individual patients' outcomes that result from the pharmacists' actions represents a significant advance in pharmacy's continuing professionalization. The provision of pharmaceutical care represents a maturation of pharmacy as a clinical profession and is a natural evolution of more mature clinical pharmacy activities of pharmacists.[14]

ASHP believes that pharmaceutical care is fundamental to the profession's purpose of helping people make the best use of medications.[15] It is a unifying concept that transcends all types of patients and all categories of pharmacists and pharmacy organizations. Pharmaceutical care is applicable and achievable by pharmacists in all practice settings. The provision of pharmaceutical care is not limited to pharmacists in inpatient, outpatient, or community settings, nor to pharmacists with certain degrees, specialty certifications, residencies, or other credentials. It is not limited to those in academic or teaching settings. Pharmaceutical care is not a matter of formal credentials or place of work. Rather, it is a matter of a direct personal, professional, responsible relationship with a patient to ensure that the patient's use of medication is optimal and leads to improvements in the patient's quality of life.

Pharmacists should commit themselves to continuous care on behalf of individual patients. They bear responsibility for ensuring that the patient's care is ongoing despite work-shift changes, weekends, and holidays. An important implication is that a pharmacist providing pharmaceutical care may need to work as a member of a team of pharmacists who provide backup care when the primary responsible pharmacist is not available. Another is that the responsible pharmacist should work to ensure that continuity of care is maintained when a patient moves from one component of a healthcare system to another (e.g., when a patient is hospitalized or discharged from a hospital to return to an ambulatory, community status). In the provision of pharmaceutical care, professional communication about the patient's needs between responsible pharmacists in each area of practice is, therefore, essential. ASHP believes that the development of recognized methods of practicing pharmaceutical care that will enhance such communication is an important priority for the profession.

Pharmaceutical care can be conceived as both a purpose for pharmacy practice and a purpose of medication use processes. That is, a fundamental professional reason that pharmacists engage in pharmacy practice should be to deliver pharmaceutical care. Furthermore, the medication use systems that pharmacists (and others) operate should be designed to support and enable the delivery of pharmaceutical care by individual pharmacists. ASHP believes that, in organized healthcare settings, pharmaceutical care can be most successfully provided when it is part of the pharmacy department's central mission and when management activity is focused on facilitating the provision of pharmaceutical care by individual pharmacists. This approach, in which empowered frontline staff provide direct care to individual patients and are supported by managers, other pharmacists, and support systems, is new for many pharmacists and managers.

An important corollary to this approach is that pharmacists providing pharmaceutical care in organized healthcare settings cannot provide such care alone. They must work in an interdependent fashion with colleagues in pharmacy and other disciplines, support systems and staff, and managers.[7] It is incumbent upon pharmacists to design work systems and practices that appropriately focus the efforts of all activities and support systems on meeting the needs of patients. Some patients will require different levels of care, and it may be useful to structure work systems in light of those differences.[16,17] ASHP believes that the provision of pharmaceutical care and the development of effective work systems to document and support it are major priorities for the profession.

In the provision of pharmaceutical care, pharmacists use their unique perspective and knowledge of medication therapy to evaluate patients' actual and potential medication-related problems. To do this, they require direct access to clinical information about individual patients. They make judgments regarding medication use and then advocate optimal medication use for individual patients in cooperation with other professionals and in consideration of their unique professional knowledge and evaluations. Pharmaceutical care includes the active participation of the patient (and designated caregivers such as family members) in matters pertinent to medication use.

The acknowledgment of pharmacists' responsibility for therapeutic outcomes resulting from their actions does not contend that pharmacists have exclusive authority for matters related to medication use. Other healthcare professionals, including physicians and nurses, have valuable and well-established, well-recognized roles in the medication use process. The pharmaceutical care concept does not diminish the roles or responsibilities of other health professionals, nor does it imply any usurping of authority by pharmacists. Pharmacists' actions in pharmaceutical care should be conducted and viewed as collaborative. The knowledge, skills, and traditions of pharmacists, however, make them legitimate leaders of efforts by healthcare teams to improve patients' medication use.

Pharmaceutical care requires a direct relationship between a pharmacist and an individual patient. Some pharmacists and other pharmacy personnel engage in clinical and product-related pharmacy activities that do not involve a direct relationship with the patient. Properly designed, these activities can be supportive of pharmaceutical care, but ASHP believes it would be confusing and counterproductive to characterize such activities as pharmaceutical care. ASHP believes that clinical and product-related pharmacy activities are essential, however, and are as important as the actions of pharmacists interacting directly with patients.

Pharmaceutical educators must teach pharmaceutical care to students.[18] Providers of continuing education should help practicing pharmacists and other pharmacy personnel understand pharmaceutical care. Students and pharmacists should be taught to conceptualize and execute responsible medication-related problem-solving on behalf of individual patients. Curricula should be designed to produce graduates with sufficient knowledge and skills to provide pharmaceutical care competently.[8,18] Initiatives are under way to bring about these changes.[8] Practicing pharmacists must commit their time as preceptors and their workplaces as teaching laboratories for the undergraduate and postgraduate education and training necessary to produce pharmacists who can provide pharmaceutical care.[8]

Research is needed to evaluate various methods and systems for the delivery of pharmaceutical care.

Pharmaceutical care represents an exciting new vision for pharmacy. ASHP hopes that all pharmacists in all practice settings share in this vision and that the pharmaceutical care concept will serve as a stimulus for them to work toward transforming the profession to actualize that vision.

References

1. Brodie DC. Is pharmaceutical education prepared to lead its profession? The Ninth Annual Rho Chi Lecture. *Rep Rho Chi.* 1973;39:6–12.

2. Brodie DC, Parish PA, Poston JW. Societal needs for drugs and drug related services. *Am J Pharm Educ.* 1980;44:276–8.

3. Hepler CD, Strand LM. Opportunities and responsibilities in pharmaceutical care. *Am J Hosp Pharm.* 1990;47:533–43.

4. Penna RP. Pharmaceutical care: pharmacy's mission for the 1990s. *Am J Hosp Pharm.* 1990;47:543–9.

5. Pierpaoli PG, Hethcox JM. Pharmaceutical care: new management and leadership imperatives. *Top Hosp Pharm Manage.* 1992;12:1–18.

6. Oddis JA. Report of the House of Delegates: June 3 and 5, 1991. *Am J Hosp Pharm.* 1991;48:1739–48.

7. American Pharmaceutical Association. An APhA white paper on the role of the pharmacist in comprehensive medication use management; the delivery of pharmaceutical care. Washington, DC: American Pharmaceutical Association; March 1992.

8. Commission to Implement Change in Pharmaceutical Education. A position paper. Entry-level education in pharmacy: a commitment to change. *AACP News.* 1991;Nov (Suppl):14.

9. Oddis JA. Report of the House of Delegates: June 1 and 3, 1992. *Am J Hosp Pharm.* 1992;49:1962–73.

10. Gouveia WA. Measuring and managing patient outcomes. *Am J Hosp Pharm.* 1992; 49:2157–8.

11. MacKeigan LD, Pathak DS. Overview of health-related quality-of-life measures. *Am J Hosp Pharm.* 1992;49:2236–45.

12. Galinsky RE, Nickman NA. Pharmacists and the mandate of pharmaceutical care. *DICP Ann Pharmacother.* 1991;21:431–4.

13. Angaran DM. Quality assurance to quality improvement: measuring and monitoring pharmaceutical care. *Am J Hosp Pharm.* 1991;48:1901–7.

14. Hepler CD. Pharmaceutical care and specialty practice. *Pharmacotherapy.* 1993; 13:64S–9S.

15. Zellmer WA. Expressing the mission of pharmacy practice. *Am J Hosp Pharm.* 1991; 48:1195. Editorial.

16. Smith WE, Benderev K. Levels of pharmaceutical care: a theoretical model. *Am J Hosp Pharm.*1991;48:540–6.

17. Strand LM, Cipolle RJ, Morley PC, et al. Levels of pharmaceutical care: a needs-based approach. *Am J Hosp Pharm.* 1991;48:547–50.

18. O'Neil EH. Health professions education for the future: schools in service to the nation. San Francisco, CA: Pew Health Profession Commission; 1993.

Originally published in Am J Hosp Pharm. *1993;50:1720–3. ©American Society of Health-System Pharmacists, Inc. All rights reserved. Reprinted with permission.*

Answers to ✓
Self Assessment Questions

Chapter 1

Question 1.1

First Patient

Without additional information it would seem that Janice is making the transition from oral medication to insulin to treat her diabetes. To help her transition smoothly and maintain tight control of her blood glucose, you may want to gather further information, including:

- Her blood glucose readings on the oral medication. Was it the optimum regimen for her?

- Her diet and exercise routines, and how well she adheres to them.

- Medication she is taking for other conditions, and how well they are controlled.

- Whether Humulin 70/30 is a good choice for tight control.

- Questions she may have about giving herself injections and other aspects of her new regime.

- Whether she has the necessary supplies and training to administer her insulin.

- If she has a clear plan for follow-up and knows what to do in the case of low blood sugars.

This case illustrates how important it is to have knowledge about the patient in order to determine if a problem exists, and if so, what that problem would be. Many patients have fractionated care either due to personal choice or because of health insurance or payment issues. In this case, if oral medications were not optimized, then insulin may not be the best choice. If Janice has uncontrolled hypothyroidism it could affect her diabetes control. A different insulin product and regimen may be necessary if we want tight blood glucose control. If Janice cannot mentally or physically administer the insulin other alternatives need to be considered.

We need to learn more about Janice's situation before assessing the appropriateness of this change in therapy. It cannot be assumed that she is ready to leave the pharmacy with the insulin and can take care of herself in a safe manner.

To prevent the problem, a pharmacist caring for this patient could have:

• Worked with Janice to maximize the outcomes from the oral medication.

• Supported her efforts to make dietary and lifestyle changes.

• Assessed her willingness to move to injections of insulin and her desire for control.

• Made recommendations to Janice's physician that might work better for her.

Second Patient

Edith's problem seems to involve the ability to take a prescribed medication or the dosage form, although it might also be an issue of the dosage form selected, and possibly of the drug itself. Assisting her with cutting the tablets would address the problem of being able to take the correct dosage, but you might want to address other possibilities, such as:

• Reviewing the new therapy.

• Doing a quick assessment of appropriateness of drug and dose.

• Making sure Edith can take it as prescribed.

In order to help Edith, we need to collect more information to determine the real problem. Perhaps more important than our duty to the patient at this point is our duty prior to filling this medication order in the first place. Should we have known that Edith had arthritis affecting her hands? This would be important for any therapies requiring dexterity and even to decide what type of caps to put on her bottles. Should we have talked with Edith before she left the pharmacy about her medicines? It would have only taken a few minutes to review the new therapy, done a quick assessment of appropriate drug and dose, and made certain that Edith would be able to take it as prescribed. Appropriate action on the part of the pharmacist could have prevented this situation from occurring once the patient got home with the medication.

To prevent the problem, a pharmacist caring for this patient could have:

• Assessed Edith's medical situation.

• Talked about what therapies would work best for her.

Third Patient

George is dealing with congestive heart failure, so we need to assess factors that can prevent him from maintaining a stable fluid and functional status. It would be important for you to know:

• George's complete medication history.

- How the medications have been used prior to this hospitalization.

- If George has experienced adverse effects from drug interaction or noncompliance with therapy.

This is example of fractionated care, where assumptions have been made by all involved that the other parties know George's entire history. In some cases the pharmacist may be the only person to know that the patient is seeking care from a variety of providers. As patients with congestive heart failure can be very hard to maintain in a stable fluid and functional status, all factors which can upset that equilibrium need to be known by those caring for these patients. It is likely that the unknown medications or some lifestyle change has caused this complication in George's condition. It could be caused by a drug's adverse effect, from a drug interaction leading to an adverse effect, or from noncompliance with therapy.

To prevent the problem, a pharmacist caring for this patient could have:

- Contacted George's community pharmacist and other prescribers.

- Made recommendations on appropriate therapy.

- Helped coordinate communication between providers.

Once a good history is known and the potential drug-related issues are identified, the pharmacist can then make recommendations to the other providers on appropriate therapy. The existence of multiple providers for a patient with a labile condition should have resulted in increased attention by the pharmacist, which then would have led to communication with the various prescribers.

Fourth Patient

Mary does not have the best dosage forms for her treatment. Some of her medicines may be crushable, but that doesn't mean the powder would be appropriate to put down a tube. Additionally, not all liquid dosage forms are good candidates for putting down a tube.

You will need to collect information about:

- Type and size of tube that Mary will be using.

- Changes that will be occurring in her drug therapy.

- What she will be using for nutrition, limitations on fluid intake, etc.

Switching medication orders between different dosage forms occurs frequently in care settings as patients' ability to swallow liquid and then solid dosage forms changes with their health status. Some medications may be discontinued and some will likely be added as she proceeds through whatever medical challenge awaits her. Once the data is collected, the pharmacist can make clear recommendations to Mary and her other providers as to how to best adjust her medicines to be given by this route.

To prevent the problem, a pharmacist caring for this patient could have:

- Planned for the change in dosage forms.

Most likely little could have been done by a pharmacist to prevent this problem, other than perhaps contributing to the effort to prevent the condition for which the tube is being placed. However, knowing the patient's medical history better would have allowed the pharmacist to proactively plan for the change in dosage forms and not wait for the patient to ask.

Question 1.2

A pharmacist may have the ability to provide excellent care to a patient, but not have the opportunity. If a pharmacist is tasked with performing duties that are not care-related he may not have time to collect information to identify problems, or he may not be in the best physical location for accessing information. If the practice is not supportive of the pharmacist performing these functions when time and place permit, he would need to fight against the system to provide this type of care. When systems are in place to support and encourage the delivery of pharmaceutical care, it then depends on the pharmacist to provide that care.

Question 1.3

Some possible ways to restate the definition of pharmaceutical care include:

- Use of patient care skills and knowledge to achieve optimal outcomes in patients' medication-related health care.

- Finding, fixing, or preventing drug therapy problems.

- The patient needs to have his or her medications reviewed and monitored to assure the best outcomes of therapy.

Note that the word "pharmacist" is never used in the above examples. A major challenge for the profession is to clearly delineate pharmacists as the health care professionals both best qualified and able to provide this type of care.

Question 1.4

Having a wide range of medications available has resulted in an overall improvement in health care outcomes over the last century. But the climate is continually changing: physicians are seeing more patients for briefer visits, health care costs are increasing, and the population is aging. Patients may have more questions about medications, but fewer opportunities to ask them. Pharmaceutical care can provide the services that physicians and the health care system cannot, and also help prevent adverse outcomes.

In addition, the use of medications in our health care system results in considerable morbidity and mortality. Health care costs associated with suboptimal prescribing of medications, inappropriate usage by patients, and adverse events associated with medications may equal that of the medications themselves. As up to one-half of these negative outcomes may be preventable, it is only logical that pharmaceutical care should be provided to patients as a way to lessen this burden on health care costs and on human suffering.

Question 1.5
Medication errors are an important cause of drug therapy problems that patients may experience. They may lead to a relatively easily identified problem or one that is difficult to discover, as the error may be difficult to recognize.

However, other drug therapy problems exist that aren't necessarily due to medication error. Problems such as the need for additional drug therapy for a new or existing medical problem, adverse drug reactions, and issues due to actions by the patients may impact the success of treatment. To have the full effect on the health of patients, the provision of pharmaceutical care goes beyond the prevention or correction of medication errors.

Question 1.6
Factors that have changed in the health care system that affect the practice of pharmacy include:

• More drugs overall, and more potent drugs are being used in the treatment of disease.

• Complex drug selection, dosage, and monitoring are necessary for many drugs.

• Patient is often further removed from the decision-making process.

• Insurance companies and pharmacy benefit managers impact medication selection and usage.

• Cost factors are becoming increasingly important.

• Care has the potential to be increasingly fragmented.

• Mail order pharmaceuticals are used by some pharmacy benefit managers.

• Prevention and control of chronic diseases have become a health priority.

• Quality and safety issues have been identified as important health care topics.

• Medication reconciliation at care transitions is mandated by accreditation agencies.

• Implementation of Medicare Part D is progressing.

- Implementation of Medication Therapy Management Services within Medicare Part D is evolving.

All of these factors would be positively impacted by more pharmacist involvement in patient care.

Chapter 2

Question 2.1
Screening questions should include the following areas:

- Results of any recent INR tests, and whether result is in the therapeutic range.

- How Mildred takes her medication, whether use is consistent with the labeled instructions, and if the instructions have been changed by the physician.

- Questions Mildred has about taking her warfarin, and whether she is confident that she is taking it correctly.

Question 2.2
The rash from lamotrigine and Red Man Syndrome represent drug therapy problems (adverse reactions caused by a drug). Poison ivy and psoriasis are disease states. However, if the patients require drug therapy, pharmacists are qualified to make this determination for self-limited conditions that may be treated over the counter (poison ivy), but not for conditions that require a physician for proper diagnosis (psoriasis).

Question 2.3
a. The patient is not having an adequate therapeutic response. A change in her medication may be beneficial.

b. The patient is bradycardic as a result of her digoxin. Decreasing the dose should resolve the problem.

c. This patient is not expected to respond to the drug therapy, since she cannot afford to fill her prescription. A change to a cheaper medication will be necessary.

d. This patient is having an inadequate therapeutic response. Adding a drug which will help prevent her asthma will be helpful.

Question 2.4
Traditional profile review or screening software is capable of finding the following problems: "dosage too low," "dosage too high," and "inappropriate compliance." Finding drug therapy problems in this fashion is generally accidental, since the pharmacist's primary concern is dispensing the prescription correctly and performing the required counseling.

Question 2.5

These drug therapy problems cannot readily be uncovered using traditional profile review and screening software: "unnecessary drug therapy," "wrong drug," "adverse drug reaction," "needs additional drug therapy." Interviewing patients or their caregivers provides essential information for pharmacists who intend to find drug therapy problems.

Question 2.6

• Gerald's need is for his drug therapy to be effective. Possible drug therapy problems include "wrong drug" or "dosage too low." Since Gerald is taking the highest dose of simvastatin we must conclude that he is on the wrong drug.

• Linda's need is for her medication to be safe. Possible drug therapy problems are "adverse drug reaction" or "dosage too high." Since 5 mg is not an excessive dose of zolpidem, her morning grogginess is best attributed to an adverse drug reaction from the zolpidem.

• Ted's need is to have no untreated indications. His drug therapy problem is "needs additional therapy."

• Louis' need is to not have any inappropriate compliance. His drug therapy problem is "inappropriate compliance."

Question 2.7

a. Since statins are contraindicated in pregnancy, the need is "safety," the drug therapy problem is "wrong drug," and the cause is "contraindication present."

b. Seriously ill patients must have their protein load tapered up slowly to avoid causing acute increases in blood urea nitrogen (BUN). The patient's need is "safety," the drug therapy problem is "adverse reaction," and the cause is "dosage increased too rapidly."

c. The need for compliance cannot be met. The drug therapy problem is "inappropriate compliance" and the cause is "cannot administer drug."

d. Chronic, persistent asthma requires the use of a preventer (e.g. a corticosteroid) in addition to a reliever like albuterol. The need is "untreated indication," the drug therapy problem is "needs additional drug therapy," and the cause is "synergistic therapy."

e. Felodipine interacts with the bioflavonoids in grapefruit juice which can result in excessive serum levels of felodipine. The need is "safety," the drug therapy problem is "dosage too high," and the cause is "drug interaction."

f. Insulin is not stable at the temperatures that can be reached in a car's glove box. The need is "effectiveness," the drug therapy problem is "dose too low," and the cause is "incorrect storage."

g. Using two drugs from the same class to treat migraine headaches is not rational drug therapy. The need is "appropriate indication," the drug therapy problem is "unnecessary drug therapy," and the cause is "duplicate therapy."

Question 2.8

a. The combination of quinidine and amiodarone may result in a serious interaction, but unless there is evidence the interaction has occurred the drug therapy problem is potential.

b. Patient appears to be using his medication as directed, but continues to have asthma symptoms. This problem is actual because he is symptomatic.

c. Patient likely needs additional drug therapy but the pharmacist is not qualified to make the medical diagnosis. Until such a diagnosis is made this problem is potential.

Question 2.9

a. Asking Dr. Lattimer if she is aware of the drug's safety profile may be interpreted as condescending or insulting. Instead Fran could tell Dr. Lattimer that she does not usually see rosuvastatin prescribed for hyperlipidemia and then ask if her patients are clinically difficult to manage. Once the conversation is started, Fran can bring up the topic of drug safety and see if Dr. Lattimer's experience with rosuvastatin is different from the safety profile suggested by the literature, and possibly offer to send Dr. Lattimer some information on the drug or suggest that another agent may be a safer initial therapy.

To educate the patient about safety issues without damaging the doctor–patient relationship, Fran could say, "Dr. Lattimer has prescribed rosuvastatin to lower your cholesterol. It's a potent drug and should be quite effective, but there may be some side effects. If you notice you are starting to retain fluid, if your eyes or skin start to turn yellow, or if your stools start to look chalky, please contact Dr. Lattimer or me immediately."

b. Letricia could begin with "As you know," which assumes knowledge on Dr. Garcia's part and is not likely to offend. Letricia can also offer to monitor the patient. She could use the following script: "Dr. Garcia, as you know, co-trimoxazole can interact with phenytoin and result in potentially dangerous phenytoin levels. Did you want me to monitor the patient for toxicity or did you intend to follow her yourself? If I find she has developed excessive drowsiness or nystagmus, I will contact you immediately."

To the patient, Letricia could say, "Dr. Garcia has prescribed an antibiotic that should clear up your infection. The antibiotic may interfere with your phenytoin therapy, but we can monitor you to ensure that nothing harmful happens. If you become excessively drowsy or if your eyes start to flicker beyond your control, please contact me or Dr. Garcia right away. It's unlikely this will occur, but the doctor and I want to be sure you know what to do."

Question 2.10

Raquel needs to assure Dr. Lipchuck that she is not making any diagnosis and that she is only screening patients to identify those who require appropriate medical follow-up. If she is trained to perform cholesterol screening, she should offer to let Dr. Lipchuck review her credentials.

Chapter 3

Question 3.1

a. Subjective: verbal histories are not always reproducible.

b. Objective: repeating the pill count should provide the same results.

c. Objective: data are reproducible and taken directly from the medical record.

d. Objective: data are in the dispensing record, but incomplete because not all the patient's medications are necessarily included.

Question 3.2

The pharmacists need to introduce the concept of a pharmacist gathering a patient history. The first pharmacist does not seek explicit patient permission to proceed; the second pharmacist does.

a. "Hi, Mrs. Tepperman. My name is Ryan and I'm a pharmacist here. I want to ensure that your medications are both safe and effective. In order to make sure your new prescription for Premarin does not have any unacceptable risks, I need to ask you a rather delicate question you may never have been asked by a pharmacist before. I promise to keep all your information confidential and will use anything you tell me only to help you manage your medications. Can you please tell me if you have ever had a hysterectomy?"

b. "Hello, Mr. Wilkens. I'm Melanie Frith and I am the pharmacist working with the doctors here. One of my jobs is to see if medications played any role in bringing you here today. I also make sure that any new medications we may put you on will not interact with medicines you were taking at home. So, is it OK with you if I ask you some questions about the medications you take? That information will help us give you the safest and most effective treatment for your chest pain. (Waits for a positive response.) Great. Have you recently taken any medication like Viagra or a similar drug?"

Question 3.3

a. Patients using more than one inhaler per month either have poor inhalation technique resulting in additional medication use, have more serious asthma than can be treated with albuterol alone, or have a compliance problem with their asthma medications. Every patient using more than one albuterol inhaler per month should be assessed for inhalation technique.

b. Patients with repeated episodes of congestive heart failure and pulmonary edema benefit from assistance with managing their medications, compliance, sodium intake, and fluid balance since all of these factors can influence disease exacerbations. Pharmacists should determine which of their patients have frequent exacerbations of congestive heart failure by reviewing their patient's profiles.

c. Elderly patients receiving poly-pharmacy are at risk for a variety of drug therapy problems, including ones related to compliance, adverse events, drug interactions, affordability, and dosage selection.

Question 3.4

a. What happened after you started taking iron tablets?

b. How many nitroglycerin pills did you have to take to get relief?

c. What other questions do you have about your diabetes medication?

d. How are you planning on taking your blood pressure medications?

e. Where else are you getting your prescriptions filled?

Question 3.5

The Public Health Service questions are best for:

• Patient counseling.

• Compliance problems.

The Basic Seven are appropriate for:

• Patients with symptoms.

• Patients with adverse effects.

• To assess "need for additional drug therapy" when the patient is complaining of symptoms.

Neither the Basic Seven nor the Public Health Service question identify "needs additional drug therapy" in asymptomatic patients.

Question 3.6

a. "What did the doctor say your blood pressure was?" or "What was the lower number when the doctor took your blood pressure?"

b. "How well are your liver and kidneys working?" or "What has the doctor told you about your liver and kidneys?"

c. "How bad is the tingling in your hands and feet?"

d. "Who of your relatives has had any heart problems?"

Question 3.7

The pharmacist must ask herself, "Did a drug cause any of these problems, or do I need a drug to fix them?" In the case of the abdominal cramps and heartburn, the answer may be "yes" because prednisone and doxycycline can cause stomach problems. For shortness of breath, the answer may also be "yes" as the patient may need additional drug therapy for his respiratory condition.

Any "yes" answer means the pharmacist must continue to gather data to identify a probable drug therapy problem.

Question 3.8

Answers a and d should be included in every history obtained by the pharmacist. As medication experts, pharmacists must know as much as possible about the patient's medication use to identify any drug therapy problems. Answers b, c, and e are useful in nearly all patients, but are vital only in patients who have disease states that are complicated by these factors.

Question 3.9

a. Subjective: patient's perception of improvements in GERD symptoms and development of any new, unexpected symptoms that could be adverse effects (e.g., headache, rash). Objective: none.

b. Subjective: patient's perception of improvements in depressive symptoms and development of any new, unexpected symptoms that could be adverse effects (e.g., insomnia, drowsiness, sexual dysfunction). Objective: none.

c. Subjective: patient's perception of any new, unexpected symptoms that could be adverse effects or complications of the disease state (e.g., rash, symptoms of hypoglycemia, foot ulcers, changes in vision). Objective: blood glucose.

Question 3.10

Since the patient is over 80, her renal and hepatic function have likely diminished, necessitating possible dosage reductions. This patient is receiving a higher dose of digoxin than would be expected for her age. The pharmacist can use demographic information to gather some focused history on the patient's digoxin use, renal function, and evidence of digoxin toxicity in order to assess her risk for a drug therapy problem.

Question 3.11

The patient is elderly and suffers from both glaucoma and Type 1 diabetes. The pharmacist must determine if any visual changes caused by either the glaucoma or the diabetes have affected the patient's ability to properly load the insulin syringe and administer her medication.

Question 3.12

The patient suffers from Type 1 diabetes. He presents new prescriptions suggestive of travel to a hot climate malaria zone, which may affect his ability to store his insulin so it remains stable. The pharmacist may also inquire if Ken will need a letter to any customs authorities describing his need for importing syringes into the country.

Question 3.13

If the pharmacist merely says "Yes" the patient is at risk for simply stopping her medication, which could result in her beginning to seize. The patient's real question is how to manage breastfeeding while taking dilantin. Asking questions about the patient's likely seizure disorder, how much medication she takes, how old the baby is, and how much the baby breastfeeds will provide information that can be used to prevent possible compliance and seizure-related problems.

Chapter 4

Question 4.1

Medication	Symptom/Indication per patient	Indication per chart
Calcium Carbonate (OTC)	brittle bones	none
EC ASA (OTC)	thin blood	none
Esomeprazole	heartburn	GERD
Nitroglycerin spray 400 mcg	chest pain	angina
Amlodipine	blood pressure	hypertension
Acetaminophen w Codeine 30 mg	foot/knee pain	osteoarthritis
Tiotropium Inhaler Capsules	asthma	none
Atenolol	blood pressure	hypertension
Nitroglycerin Patch	chest pain	angina
Ramipril	blood pressure	hypertension
Acetaminophen (OTC)	pain	osteoarthritis
None	Fatigue	none
None	None	Type 2 Diabetes

Mrs. Rifkin can state an indication for why she is taking calcium carbonate, tiotropium, and EC ASA, but there is no corresponding diagnosis in the patient's medical record to support her use of these medications.

There is no corresponding diagnosis of fatigue in the medical record, nor is Mrs. Rifkin taking any medication to treat fatigue. She is identified as being diabetic, but is not taking any medication for it. For the remaining medications, the indication stated by the patient is similar to that provided in the medical record.

All conditions except fatigue and diabetes are being managed; all medications except calcium carbonate, EC ASA, and tiotropium appear to be managing a condition. We cannot conclude if there are or are not any drug therapy problems. Next steps include obtaining more information on use of calcium carbonate, tiotropium, and EC ASA.

Similarly, her fatigue and diabetes must be explored. Could a medication have caused them or is a medication needed to treat them?

Question 4.2

Condition as per patient and/or chart	Treatment
Angina	Nitroglycerin spray and patch
Type 2 Diabetes	Diet
Gastro-esophageal reflux disease (GERD)	Esomeprazole
Hypertension	Amlodipine, atenolol, ramipril
Osteoarthritis with right total knee replacement	Acetaminophen w Codeine, Acetaminophen
Fatigue	None

Here we can conclude that Mrs. Rifkin is receiving therapy for her diabetes, which is controlled with diet. The fatigue remains an issue. It is not being treated with drug or non-drug therapy, and it is not clear at this point if therapy is indicated. Fatigue, however, is a well recognized adverse effect of atenolol and both onset and duration of her fatigue are consistent with atenolol administration. We cannot conclude that Mrs. Rifkin has any untreated indications, but the connection between fatigue and atenolol is a working hypothesis.

Question 4.3

Medication	Symptom/Indication per patient	Indication per chart
Calcium Carbonate (OTC)	brittle bones	none
EC ASA (OTC)	thin blood	none
Esomeprazole	heartburn	GERD
Nitroglycerin spray 400 mcg	chest pain	angina
Amlodipine	blood pressure	hypertension
Acetaminophen w Codeine 30 mg	foot/knee pain	osteoarthritis
Tiotropium Inhaler Capsules	asthma	none
Atenolol	blood pressure	hypertension
Nitroglycerin Patch	chest pain	angina
Ramipril	blood pressure	hypertension
Acetaminophen (OTC)	pain	osteoarthritis

Most of Mrs. Rifkin's medications appear to be linked to an appropriate indication. Calcium carbonate is present although there is nothing in the patient's chart to support a diagnosis of osteoporosis. Yet Mrs. Rifkin's use of calcium seems reasonable; she is post menopausal and ensuring adequate calcium intake is necessary to maintain bone health.

There is nothing in the chart to definitively support the use of EC ASA, but Mrs. Rifkin does have a history of angina and EC ASA may be justifiable as primary prevention against myocardial infarction. Since the medication was purchased as a nonprescription, it is possible that Dr. Hale is unaware of its use. At the very least, the pharmacist needs to confirm with the physician that the patient should be on EC ASA.

Mrs. Rifkin claims to have asthma, but there is nothing in the medical record to support that statement. Plus tiotropium is more appropriately used for chronic obstructive pulmonary disease (COPD) than asthma. Since tiotropium requires a prescription it is likely that Dr. Hale is aware of its use and that the lack of a documented indication is simply an oversight, but we need to confirm its appropriateness.

Question 4.4

Using the assessment questions in Table 4-1, we arrive at the following answers:

Question	Answer
Any untreated indications?	Need more information to assess (fatigue) but may be an adverse reaction of atenolol.
Need for synergistic therapy?	Yes. Hypertension already being treated with synergistic combination therapy.
Need for prophylactic therapy?	No evidence to suggest so.
Is each medication correlated with a condition?	Yes according to patient. No according to chart.
Is patient misusing medication?	No evidence to suggest so.
Is non-drug therapy preferable?	Already managing diabetes this way.
Inappropriate duplicate therapy?	No evidence to suggest so.
Drugs being used to treat adverse effects?	No evidence to suggest so.

We can conclude:

- We need to continue exploring the etiology and treatment of Mrs. Rifkin's fatigue although an adverse effect of atenolol appears to be a reasonable explanation. It does not appear she has any untreated indications.

- All medications appear to have an appropriate indication, but we need to confirm this with Dr. Hale for the EC ASA and tiotropium. Until then, these will be considered as potential drug therapy problems of unnecessary drug indication caused by no medical indication.

Question 4.5

Possible dosage- and dosage-schedule-related problems can be identified for the following medications:

- Calcium carbonate: Mrs. Rifkin is taking 1500 mg of calcium carbonate daily, equivalent to 600 mg of elemental calcium. This is only half the 1200 mg of elemental calcium recommended as the daily requirement of a post menopausal female. This is an actual drug therapy problem unless subsequent information indicates she consumes large amounts of calcium-rich foods.

- Esomeprazole: Although 40 mg of esomeprazole daily may be required for severe GERD that does not respond to lower doses, most patients can be managed with 20 mg per day. This seems to be a potential drug therapy problem.

- Acetaminophen: Mrs. Rifkin can potentially take her nonprescription acetaminophen as 1 g every 4 hours or 6 g per day. In addition, she has a prescription for acetaminophen with codeine which provides another 500 mg per tablet. Consequently, Mrs. Rifkin's total potential exposure to acetaminophen is over 6 g per day. This dose is well recognized to be potentially hepatotoxic.

Mrs. Rifkin appears to have three drug therapy problems related to drug dosage or schedule:

- Dosage of calcium too low (actual).

- Dosage of esomeprazole too high (potential).

- Dosage/dosage interval of acetaminophen too high (potential).

These drug therapy problems are not based on patient-specific data. Without having more dietary information, we cannot be certain that the dose of calcium is too low. Mrs. Rifkin does not complain of any adverse effects of esomeprazole. Neither does she complain of ongoing GERD symptoms suggestive of a dosing problem with her medication. The best we can conclude is that, using non-patient-specific information, Mrs. Rifkin may have the drug therapy problem of too high a dosage of esomeprazole. According to the patient, Mrs. Rifkin only takes her acetaminophen (both plain and with codeine) about once per week. Based on her actual drug intake, any dosage-related problems with acetaminophen are only potential since she has no evidence of hepatic injury.

Question 4.6
Nearly all of Mrs. Rifkin's medical conditions are chronic and long-term therapy is indicated. Although many patients with GERD require ongoing therapy, the package insert for esomeprazole suggests that patients should be tried on short-term therapy first. Thus, there is a potential drug therapy problem (dosage too high) related to the duration of esomeprazole therapy. Again, this problem is not based on any patient-specific information, only on the drug literature.

Question 4.7
Most of Mrs. Rifkin's medications are oral dosage forms with the exception of the nitroglycerin spray and patch and the tiotropium which is a capsule for oral inhalation. The esomeprazole is a sustained release dosage form. There is no evidence to suggest there is any drug therapy problem related to dosage form.

Question 4.8
Most of Mrs. Rifkin's medication choices seem appropriate for her medical conditions. However, EC ASA may be relatively contraindicated due to her history of GERD as may atenolol if she does have asthma. She does not voice any complaints about her response to drug therapy and her laboratory tests do not indicate any therapeutic failures, but the following conditions present opportunities for improvement.

- Osteoporosis: A bisphosphonate added to the calcium may be more effective therapy than calcium alone because bisphosphonates prevent bone resorption while calcium alone does not.

- GERD: Esomeprazole is no more effective for most cases of GERD than omeprazole, and it is also more expensive because it is not available generically. Her use of EC ASA may also be exacerbating her GERD symptoms.

- Asthma: There may be more effective medication than tiotropium available since this agent is generally used for bronchospasm associated with chronic obstructive pulmonary disease, rather than asthma. Atenolol may not be the best choice for asthma.

It is important to confirm the indications for calcium and tiotropium before concluding they are the wrong medications, but if they are correct, the potential drug therapy problem of wrong drug due to no medical indication exists. Mrs. Rifkin has adequate insurance, so the cost of esomeprazole does not seem to be an issue. Nevertheless, there is no advantage to using the more expensive agent and the problem of "wrong drug" due to more effective (i.e., cheaper) medication available does seem to be a reasonable conclusion. If the EC ASA is worsening her GERD symptoms, or atenolol is worsening possible asthma that relative contraindication would also constitute a potential drug therapy problem of "wrong drug" caused by contraindication present. All five of these drug therapy problems are potential, based more upon literature information than patient-specific data.

Question 4.9

According to her history, Mrs. Rifkin claims to have no problems with medication compliance. But a check of the refill dates shows that she is approximately one week later refilling her atenolol than she is for refilling her other antihypertensive medications (which are all refilled on the same date). A potential drug therapy problem of inappropriate compliance with atenolol is a plausible conclusion, but the evidence is weak and the cause of the problem is not apparent.

Question 4.10

Fatigue is the only patient complaint that has not already been diagnosed by Dr. Hale. Atenolol remains a logical explanation for the fatigue. Mrs. Rifkin is not taking any medications to which she has a documented allergy. There is no evidence of any drug interactions.

Question 4.11

Actual problems:

- Adverse drug reaction caused by undesirable effect caused by atenolol.

- "Dosage too low" caused by wrong dosage for calcium carbonate.

Potential problems:

- "Dosage too high" caused by wrong dosage for esomeprazole and acetaminophen. In addition, same problem caused by duration inappropriate for esomeprazole.

- "Wrong drug" caused by more effective drug therapy available for esomeprazole.

- "Wrong drug" caused by contraindication present for EC ASA.

- "Needs additional drug therapy" caused by need for synergistic therapy with calcium and a biphosphonate.

Potential problems pending additional information from Dr. Hale or Mrs. Rifkin:

- "No indication" caused by no medical indication for EC ASA and tiotropium.

- "Inappropriate compliance" for atenolol. Cause cannot be identified.

- "Wrong drug" caused by more effective drug therapy available for tiotropium.

- "Wrong drug" caused by contraindication present for atenolol in asthma.

It seems that all problems have been identified, though it is unlikely that all of them would truly be considered drug therapy problems. For example, esomeprazole is identified as having too high a dose, too long a duration of therapy, and being the wrong drug. If it is genuinely the wrong drug (and presumably therapy will be changed) then the dose and duration of therapy don't really matter. In other cases (e.g., no indication for tiotropium) once we can clarify the drug's indication with Dr. Hale, it is likely that this will turn out not to be a drug therapy problem, but just a missing piece of data.

Chapter 5

Question 5.1
Actual problems: Both exist, automatically meriting the pharmacist's further attention, and must be included on a revised list.

Potential problems: Acetaminophen can be removed (a too high dose seems unlikely since the patient takes it infrequently). Esomeprazole "duration inappropriate" can be removed (few patients respond well to only a short course of a proton pump inhibitor. Most patients end up on long-term therapy). Esomeprazole "dosage too high" is irrelevant if "wrong drug" is retained since a more effective alternative is available. Adding additional therapy to calcium is plausible, so "needs additional drug therapy" will be retained. Nothing in Mrs. Rifkin's history or interview suggests that the EC ASA is causing her any significant problems, so it can be deleted.

Pending potential problems: Lack of indication for the EC ASA and tiotropium can be readily resolved by asking the physician, so these problems can be removed. Before calling the compliance problem with atenolol an issue, more information is required. It can be dropped.

Without knowing the physician's indication for tiotropium, it is difficult to determine if it is the wrong drug, so this problem can also be removed as can contraindication with atenolol until a diagnosis of asthma is confirmed.

Mrs. Rifkin's Revised Drug Therapy Problem List

Actual problems:

- "Adverse drug reaction" caused by undesirable effect caused by atenolol.

- "Dosage too low" caused by wrong dosage for calcium carbonate.

    Potential problems:

- "Needs additional drug therapy" caused by need for synergistic therapy with calcium and a biphosphonate.

- "Wrong drug" caused by more effective drug therapy available for esomeprazole.

Question 5.2
- Adverse effect of atenolol: acute, not serious, Priority II.

- Dosage too low of calcium: not acute, not serious, Priority III.

- Needs additional drug therapy (Calcium): not acute, not serious, Priority III.

- Wrong drug (esomeprazole): not acute, not serious, Priority III.

Question 5.3
a. The patient will no longer complain of more migraine headaches than he is willing to tolerate.

b. The patient will demonstrate an understanding of why he must stop smoking and demonstrate an acceptance of enrolling in a smoking cessation program.

c. The goal is outside the pharmacist's scope of practice. It should not be reworded but left to a qualified physician.

Question 5.4
a. This is a plan since the pharmacist or the physician will start the patient on enalapril. It should be reworded as, "The patient will begin taking enalapril 5 mg daily for hypertension," or "The patient's blood pressure will be adequately controlled on enalapril 5 mg qd."

b. This is a plan since the pharmacist or physician is changing the medication. It should be reworded as, "The patient will start taking atorvastatin 20 mg in place of pravastatin 20 mg," or "The patient will lower his total cholesterol to < 200 mg/dL on atorvastatin 20 mg qd."

c. This is a goal since the patient is the one who will be taking the blood pressure.

d. This is a plan since the pharmacist will enroll the patient. It should be reworded to, "The patient will enroll in our asthma management program."

Question 5.5

a. The patient will experience resolution of her fatigue to her satisfaction without a commensurate change in blood pressure or increased incidence of angina.

b. Can combine this goal statement with (c).

c. Combining (b) and (c), The patient will receive the recommended daily allowance of calcium and begin additional therapy with a bisphosphonate. She will avoid signs and symptoms of osteoporosis as well as adverse effects of her calcium and bisphosphonate therapy.

d. The patient will receive more effective (or more cost-effective) therapy for her GERD, have resolution of GERD symptoms, and not experience adverse effects caused by her GERD therapy.

Question 5.6

a. Decrease dose of atenolol to 25 mg qd; change atenolol to chlorthalidone 25 mg po qd; change atenolol to prazosin 1 mg qd.

b. Increase calcium to calcium carbonate 1500 mg bid with meals; change calcium to calcium citrate 950 mg 2 tablets tid with meals.

c. Add alendronate 35 mg q weekly; add risedronate 35 mg weekly; add ibandronate 150 mg q monthly.

d. Change esomeprazole to generic omeprazole 20 mg qd; change esomeprazole to lansoprazole 15 mg qd.

Question 5.7

The fatigue is likely to resolve, but if the atenolol is discontinued and no alternative therapy is started she may have a clinical deterioration in her angina and hypertension.

Question 5.8

A patient-focused intervention for the first drug therapy problem would involve significant patient education on sleep hygiene. Topics such as caffeine intake, exercise, bed times, sleeping conditions in the bedroom, reading or watching television in bed, daytime naps, etc. would be discussed.

A patient-focused intervention for the calcium dosage would involve obtaining a detailed dietary history from Mrs. Rifkin and determining her dietary intake. The pharmacist would develop a plan for Mrs. Rifkin so that her intake from both the calcium carbonate tablets and her diet reaches her recommended daily allowance for calcium.

Question 5.9

a. Decrease atenolol dosage to 25 mg qd for one week. Monitor response in 7 days for changes in fatigue, blood pressure, and angina.

b. Increase calcium carbonate dosage to 1500 mg (equivalent to 600 mg elemental calcium) twice daily and assess patient's tolerance in 7 days.

Question 5.10

Drug-focused aspects:

Decrease atenolol to 25 mg qd. This is the most rational choice. Mrs. Rifkin is already on the medication so she will not need to get a new prescription but can take a half tablet of her existing supply. Other than the fatigue it causes no other problems and her hypertension and angina seem already well controlled on atenolol. Neither chlorthalidone nor prazosin would effectively treat her angina.

Increase calcium carbonate to 1500 mg twice daily. This will provide Mrs. Rifkin with the recommended 1200 mg of calcium daily. She is already taking this form of calcium and so will not need to purchase a new product. She can take this as 750 mg tablets, two tablets twice daily with meals which is more likely to promote compliance than the three times a day dosage schedule of calcium citrate. However, it may have a higher incidence of gastric intolerance than calcium citrate.

Add risedronate 35 mg weekly. All three of these options are plausible. The best choice will account for the drug's cost, the patient's insurance coverage and the patient's preference for taking medication weekly versus monthly. Absent such information, risedronate is a reasonable choice.

Change esomeprazole to omeprazole 20 mg daily. Omeprazole would be expected to be equally effective, but less expensive. Depending on the patient's insurance, the nonprescription dosage form is also an option. Lansoprazole is clinically equivalent to either alternative, but has no particular clinical or financial advantage.

Patient-focused aspects: Ensure that Mrs. Rifkin agrees with all aspects of the care plan. Ensure that she has 25 mg atenolol tablets or knows how to break 50 mg tablets and that she will continue to take the atenolol once daily. Ensure that she has calcium carbonate 750 mg tablets and knows how to take two tablets twice daily with meals. Ensure she has a new prescription for risedronate and understands how to take the medication properly. Ensure that she either has a new prescription for omeprazole 20 mg or has purchased the nonprescription product and knows how to take the medication. Ensure she is aware of all adverse effects of all medications and knows whom to contact should they occur. Obtain Mrs. Rifkin's approval for the monitoring plan (see below) and confirm that she will return to the correct place at the correct time for necessary follow-up.

Monitoring plan:

Atenolol: follow up in the pharmacy in 1 week, then in 1 month and then quarterly. Monitor patient's subjective complaints of fatigue and frequency of angina. Measure blood pressure at each visit. Monitor for patient compliance and statements of new problems or complaints. Contact physician if hypertension or angina not controlled on 25 mg qd or if fatigue does not respond to dosage decrease.

Calcium: follow up in the pharmacy in 1 week, then in 1 month and then quarterly. Monitor for patient complaints of gastric upset. Monitor for compliance and statements of new problems or complaints. Monitor dietary calcium intake.

Risedronate: follow up in the pharmacy in 1 week, then in 1 month and then quarterly. Monitor that patient is taking medication correctly (empty stomach, full glass of water, remaining upright). Monitor for adverse effects such as headache, rash, diarrhea, arthralgia, gastric intolerance, etc., and contact physician if they occur. Monitor for compliance and statements of new problems or complaints. Suggest physician obtain baseline bone density and monitor annually.

Omeprazole follow up in the pharmacy in 1 week, then in 1 month and then quarterly. Monitor for GERD symptoms. Contact physician if inadequate therapeutic response to new drug. Monitor for compliance and statements of new problems or complaints.

Question 5.11
Dear Dr. Hale:

I recently reviewed Mrs. Annette Rifkin's drug therapy at your request. After interviewing Mrs. Rifkin and reviewing her medication profile and medical record, I offer the following concerns about her response to her medication.

She complains of morning fatigue that resolves by mid-afternoon most days. This is consistent with both the side effect profile and pharmacokinetics of atenolol.

Her nonprescription calcium carbonate dosage is 1500 mg daily. This is equivalent to 600 mg of elemental calcium which is only half of her requirements to maintain bone health. She may also benefit from the addition of a bisphosphonate to her calcium therapy.

Esomeprazole offers no clinical or therapeutic advantage over generic omeprazole and is considerably more expensive.

I would offer the following suggestions for your consideration.

Please consider decreasing the atenolol dose to 25 mg qd. I will monitor Mrs. Rifkin's fatigue as well as her blood pressure and complaints of angina and inform you of any clinical changes immediately.

I have instructed Mrs. Rifkin to begin taking calcium carbonate 1500 mg twice daily with meals and she agrees. You may wish to consider adding risedronate 35 mg once weekly so as to maximize her response to calcium therapy. Please consider also obtaining a baseline bone density screening so that we can monitor her response properly. I will check with Mrs. Rifkin regularly to monitor how well she is tolerating the increased calcium and the risedronate therapy.

Please consider switching the esomeprazole to generic omeprazole 20 mg daily. I will monitor Mrs. Rifkin's response and if her GERD worsens, will inform you immediately.

I hope you will find these recommendations helpful and realize you may have additional information about the patient that could render them clinically inappropriate.

Thank you for allowing me to assist in the care of this patient and feel free to contact me at 555-1234 if you have any questions.

Sincerely
David Rice, PharmD
Clinical Pharmacist

Chapter 6

Question 6.1
Patient care documentation:

- Creates a written record of care provided by the pharmacist.

- Communicates patient and care plan information.

- Assists the provider in providing care to the patient in the future.

- Provides a legal record of care for auditing by third parties or for medical and legal purposes.

Question 6.2
Recording information during the interview is (in most circumstances) collecting data, which is necessary for the identification and resolution of problems but does not equate to the provision of care. Care documentation includes not only the necessary data, but also the pharmacist's evaluation of that data, the plan to address any problems identified, and the monitoring plan to determine the success of the plan in correcting any problems.

Question 6.3

Basic components of a problem-oriented patient record include:

- A problem list (including medical problems, medications, medication allergies, and drug therapy problems) which serves as an index for the chart.

- Problem-oriented notes in chronological order.

- Various flow sheets or patient/disease specific data sheets.

- Laboratory, correspondence, or other relevant sections.

Question 6.4

Information obtained from or about the patient during data collection is included in the Subjective or Objective sections of the note. Results of the data evaluation process are documented in the Assessment section. Patient care plan development, both the therapeutic intervention and the monitoring process, is documented in the Plan section.

Question 6.5

Jane's Chart 08/30/06

Inappropriate compliance: patient taking over the prescribed amount of Imitrex.
Inappropriate compliance: patient discontinued propranolol on own.
Drug needed for untreated indication: need for migraine prophylaxis.

S: Jane presented today for a refill of her Imitrex 100 mg # 20. She states she takes three per day for the treatment of headaches, although her prescription is for one tablet, to be repeated in 2 hours if no relief, max of two per day. She has been doing this for the last two weeks. This corresponds to when she stopped her propranolol 20 mg BID abruptly due to feeling it was ineffective and giving her nightmares.

O: Refill history supports patient's history of medication use.

A: Patient is overusing her migraine acute treatment medication, possibly as a result of stopping her prophylaxis treatment. She needs effective preventative treatment to avoid excessive use of abortive therapy.

P: Instructed Jane to use no more than 2 of the Imitrex 100 mg tablets daily. I called Dr. Jones to inform him of the lack of success of propranolol, possible ADR and patient's noncompliance. I recommended desipramine 25 mg at HS #30, Dr. agreed and order transcribed. I instructed Jane to not discontinue new med without first discussing with Dr. Jones or myself.

F/U: Call patient in one week, assess for decreased frequency of migraines (goal <1/week), utilization of Imitrex, tolerability of desipramine. Transmit information collected to Dr. Jones.

Joe Pharmacist

Question 6.6

Follow-up documentation assures that the intervention made by the pharmacist has the intended outcome, and is part of providing responsible care to the patient. Without it, the pharmacist would not know if a drug therapy problem remains uncorrected or if a new drug therapy problem developed (either due to the actions of the pharmacist or independent of those actions). If this process is not documented, it is unlikely the pharmacist would remember what he needs to do when he next interacts with the patient.

When a system is put into place to make sure the monitoring is completed, therapy can be adjusted and outcomes can move closer to being achieved. Once the monitoring is completed, documenting the status of the patient and the outcome of the existing plan establishes a marker in the patient record to which future care can be compared.

Chapter 7

Answers for Sally's Case

1. First, clarify Sally's request. Which of the inhalers does she really want? Depending on her response, you need to know how she has been using the inhalers, her current level of asthma symptomatology, and how she came to be on the medications she is currently taking. It will be important to establish which physician has primary responsibility for treatment of her asthma. (Sally should be able to provide answers to all of these questions.)

In addition, her refill records could be useful to validate her history. If the pharmacy has any previous care records on Sally, they might also be helpful in clarifying the current situation.

2. a. Unnecessary drug therapy: duplicate inhaled steroid prescriptions (actual, Priority 3).

b. Dosage too high: dose of salmeterol is twice normal due to 2 prescriptions (actual, Priority 3).

c. Inappropriate compliance: patient does not understand instructions (actual, Priority 3).

3. Asthma: Prevent exacerbations of asthma as measured by no unscheduled physician visits or emergency room visits and no limitations in normal activities.

4. Contact prescribers to determine desired regimen. Recommend one inhaled steroid, with or without a long-acting sympathomimetic and one rescue inhaler.

a. Discontinue the Azmacort inhaler, discontinue the Advair inhaler.

b. Discontinue the Serevent inhaler, discontinue the Advair inhaler.

c. Clarify the correct medications and appropriate use with patient verbally, write out appropriate regimen on a daily schedule with medication names, and provide descriptions or pictures of inhalers.

5. Therapeutic plan: Contact physician to inform her of current medication usage and recommend simplification of regimen by discontinuing the Advair. Assess inhaler technique. Counsel patient on appropriate inhalers to use; provide written directions as well. Contact the patient in 1 week, review medication use, and determine success in preventing asthma symptoms. Review use and therapy outcomes at each refill opportunity.

6. Implementation Plan: Contact physician's office to obtain order clarification and new prescriptions as necessary. Counsel the patient at this time and at follow-up opportunities to assure continued appropriate use.

7. Sally Strathclyde 10/23/06
   Unnecessary drug therapy: duplicate inhaled steroid prescriptions.
   Dosage too high: dose of salmeterol is twice normal due to two prescriptions.
   Inappropriate compliance: patient does not understand instructions.

S: Sally presents to the pharmacy today wanting to get all four of her inhalers refilled. These include Advair 250/50 one puff BID, Serevent 1 puff BID, Azmacort 4 puffs BID, and albuterol 2 puffs q 4 hours prn (uses once/month). She uses the three maintenance inhalers on a daily basis. She doesn't know the names of the inhalers or their purpose. She states her asthma control is very good on the current regimen.

O: none.

A: Current regimen has duplication of inhaled steroid therapy and salmeterol therapy. This has been contributed to by having two prescribers and Sally not knowing the purpose of her medications.

P: Dr. Jones was notified of the duplication issues. She agreed to suggestion that we discontinue the Advair. New orders were written to continue only the Azmacort 4 puffs BID and the Serevent one puff BID as maintenance meds, with Albuterol 2 puffs Q 4 hours prn as a rescue inhaler.

Sally agreed to throw away the Advair she had at home. She was counseled on use for each inhaler. Changes in regimen were explained to Sally, with written instructions provided along with purpose of each inhaler. Observed her inhaler technique, which was judged to be good.

F/U: Call Sally in one week at home to review how she is currently using her inhalers. Assess her knowledge about purpose of each inhaler and also continued prevention of asthma symptoms. Continue to review use and asthma symptom control at each refill. If she remains asymptomatic for several months, consider recommending elimination of the salmeterol.

Heather Price, PharmD

Answers for James' Case

1. James is here for a check of his lipids, so we need to find out why he wants this done. If he has had levels done in the past, what were they? Is he currently on drug treatment or a lifestyle modification program to address his lipid levels? What other risk factors does he have in addition to hypertension? James should be able to help you with much of this information. You might need to contact a laboratory or a physician's office to get previous laboratory values.

2. a. Dose too low: lisinopril dose should be increased to lower BP (actual, Priority 1).

   b. Needs additional drug therapy: untreated condition, hyperlipidemia (actual, Priority 2).

3. a. Hypertension, slow progression of cardiovascular complications by reducing BP to < 140/90.

   b. Hyperlipidemia, slow progression of cardiovascular complications by reducing lipids to TC < 200, LDL < 100, TG < 150 and increasing HDL > 40.

4. a. Increase dose of lisinopril to 20 mg per day, increase dose of Toprol XL to 100 mg per day.

   b. Continue dietary changes with no added drug therapy, slowly titrate niacin up to 2000 mg/day, start lovastatin 20 mg per day, start Lipitor 10 mg per day.

5. Therapeutic plan
   a. Increase the dose of lisinopril to 20 mg per day. Although pulse is not low, lipid neutral effects of ACEI and dosing range preferred. Recheck BP beginning in 1 week, check several times over the next 2 weeks. Assess for orthostasis, cough, and other complaints after dosage increase.

   b. Lipitor 10 mg daily. James has need for 50 mg/dL decrease in LDL and increase in HDL. This will require moderately potent statin in addition to lifestyle changes. Given family history and hypertension probably best to initiate drug therapy. Recheck lipids in 3 months.

6. Implementation Plan:
   a. Contact primary care physician with BP history from pharmacy, recommend change in therapy to increase lisinopril dose, and inform of ability to follow up with BP readings in the pharmacy. Obtain new prescription.

   b. Report lipid results to physician's office. Recommend the initiation of therapy as patient has maximized lifestyle modification. Obtain new prescription.

7. James Olson
   08/06/06 Dose too low: lisinopril dose should be increased to lower BP.

S: James came in today to have his fasting lipid panel checked. He has been making dietary and exercise modification since being told his cholesterol was high 9 months ago. First diagnosed with hypertension about 3 years ago. Has been on Toprol XL 50 mg per day and lisinopril 10 mg daily since then. He states he takes these daily and this is supported by refill records. He has had several blood pressures taken in the pharmacy the last 2 months as he has focused on improving his health.

O:	BP	Date	Pulse
	140/100	today	70
	144/102	7/5/this year	68
	140/104	6/15/this year	72

A: His dose of lisinopril should be increased to further reduce his blood pressure.

P: I called Dr. Jones' office to inform them of the repeated elevated blood pressure readings from the pharmacy and suggested that we increase the lisinopril to 20 mg/day. Told the office we could follow up with BP readings after the change. Dr. Jones agreed but wants to see James in her office in one month. New Rx received and filled. Counseled James on increasing the dose of lisinopril and instructed him to call Dr. Jones' office for an appointment.

F/U: Agreed with James that he will come into the pharmacy for at least three BP readings beginning one week from now. Assess BP control with values < 140/90, for symptoms of orthostasis, cough or other complaints at each BP visit. Communicate findings to Dr. Jones' office after three values obtained.

Phillip Isaacs, PharmD

08/06/this year Needs additional drug therapy: untreated condition, hyperlipidemia.

S: James came in today to have his fasting lipid panel checked. He is following up on his progress after making dietary and exercise changes per his physician's recommendation. Last seen by physician 9 months ago, when he was told his cholesterol was "high." His next visit with the physician is "not for a while." He has eliminated added salt and high amounts of fat from his diet, and is eating more fish and chicken. He is exercising twice a week, but hopes to increase this, has been unsuccessful at this in past. He has nearly stopped smoking, is down to 3 cigarettes per day from 1 ppd. Hopes to stop for good in next 30 days. His Father had an MI at 57 y.o. and an uncle died of an MI at 37 y.o.

O: Fasting lipid profile today in pharmacy: TC 209, HDL 33, LDL 150, TG 133.

A: Lipid values not at goal after 9 months of lifestyle modifications. Given patient's risk factors feel that drug therapy is indicated.

P: I called Dr. Jones' office with fasting lipid panel results. Recommended that drug therapy is indicated at this time and suggested Lipitor 10 mg daily to start therapy. Physician wants to see patient for additional assessment and baseline laboratories before initiating treatment. I counseled patient that lipid values were not at goal and that Dr. Jones wanted to see him prior to making changes in the plan. I reinforced James' progress with lifestyle modifications and encourage further exercise if possible. James agreed to make appointment with physician.

F/U: Discuss outcome of physician visit with James at upcoming BP visits. Continue to reinforce lifestyle changes. Counsel as appropriate if medication initiated.

Phillip Isaacs, PharmD

Chapter 8

Answers for Tommy's Case

1.a. Information from the chart: history of present illness; description of hospital course; full medication history; vital signs; results of physician's physical examination; culture and sensitivity report; laboratory parameters for infection (white blood cell count with differential, erythrocyte sedimentation rate); radiology reports; kidney and liver function tests; relevant past medical history pertinent to infection or medication use.

b. Information from Tommy/mother: subjective response to antibiotic therapy; subjective reports of foot pain; subjective reports of perceived adverse drug reactions; social history that may affect home medication administration; any history of medication compliance problems; drug samples, nonprescription medications, nutritional supplements, and herbal products used.

2.a. Dosage too low: duration inappropriate of ceftazidime (actual problem, serious and acute, Priority 1).

b. Needs additional drug therapy: synergistic therapy preferred with ceftazidime (actual problem, serious and acute, Priority 1).

c. Needs additional drug therapy: untreated indication of pain (actual problem; acute, not serious; Priority 2).

3.a. Duration of therapy of ceftazidime inappropriate: Since problems a and b both result from the same medical problem, goal statements can be combined into one statement because we are choosing drug therapy for the same condition and want the same clinical outcome for both drug therapy problems. A reasonable goal would be: "The patient's infection will resolve based on signs (WBC count, cultures, radiological assessment) and symptoms (pain, fever) without drug-related complications."

b. Needs additional synergistic drug therapy: see above.

c. Untreated indication of pain: Patient will express adequate relief of his pain and the ability to engage in activities of daily living without complaining of adverse effects such as unacceptable sedation or constipation.

4. a. Duration of therapy of ceftazidime inappropriate: increase duration of ceftazidime therapy to 4 weeks; or increase duration of ceftazidime therapy to 6 weeks.

b. Needs additional synergistic drug therapy: add tobramycin 2 mg/kg IV q8h x 2 weeks; or add ciprofloxacin 250 mg po q12h x 2 weeks.

c. Untreated indication of pain: add ibuprofen suspension 20 mg/mL 10mL po q6-8h prn; or add acetaminophen plus codeine 120/12 mg/5 mL syrup 10mL po q4-6h prn.

5. a. Antibiotic therapy: ceftazidime 1g iv q8h x 4 weeks plus tobramycin 50mg iv q8h x 2 weeks.

b. Pain therapy: ibuprofen suspension 10mL po q6-8h prn pain.

c. Monitoring: vital signs daily x 1 week; subjective response to antibiotics and analgesics; tobramycin serum levels—target peak 5 mcg/mL, trough < 2mcg/mL monitored twice weekly; white blood cell and differential count twice weekly; BUN and creatinine twice weekly; antibiotic adverse effects—diarrhea, rash, ototoxicity; ibuprofen adverse effects— gastric upset.

d. Rationale: minimum 4 week course of therapy indicated. If inadequate response after 4 weeks, can increase to 6 week course of therapy. Two week course of synergistic therapy indicated. Synergy with aminoglycosides well established. Quinolones not drug of choice in children due to effect on cartilage. Ibuprofen less likely to cause constipation or sedation than opiates and available OTC.

6. Implementation will require cooperation of both Tommy's mother and the prescribing physician's assistant. Mother will need to be counseled on the appropriate product to purchase, how to determine if Tommy requires analgesia, how much medication to give, how to measure a dose appropriately, and side effects to monitor for. The physician's assistant will need to approve the proposed changes in Tommy's discharge medication and the monitoring plan. She will also have to rewrite the discharge prescriptions to reflect the changes in therapy.

7. Tommy Lohse 7/10/this year
Duration of therapy of ceftazidime inappropriate.
Needs additional synergistic drug therapy: untreated indication of pain.

S: Pharmacist requested to perform discharge counseling for this 7-year-old boy admitted for surgical debridement and antibiotic therapy of Pseudomonas aeruginosa-related osteomyelitis of right great toe. Proposed discharge medications: ceftazidime 1g iv q8h and heparin flush via PICC line x 2 weeks. During counseling, patient complained of moderate foot pain.

O: Pseudomonas susceptible to imipenem, meropenem, ceftazidime, cefipime, tobramycin and ciprofloxacin. WBC today 10,400. 64% neutrophils. Temp 36.9.

A: Recommended course of therapy for osteomyelitis would be a 4 to 6 week course of antibiotics with a synergistic combination for the first 2 weeks. Patient will also require analgesia for the first few days after discharge.

P: Suggested to mother to give Tommy ibuprofen suspension 10mL po q6-8h prn pain. Counseled on appropriate administration. Mother agrees and understands. Will purchase medication after discharge. Suggested to PA Nguyen to extend ceftazidime therapy to 4 week course and to add tobramycin 50 mg iv q8h x first 2 weeks. Suggest target peak and trough tobramycin 5 and <2 mcg/mL and to follow tobramycin levels, CBC and differential and BUN/creatinine twice weekly for duration of therapy. PA agrees. Discharge orders rewritten to include new orders. I will follow up with patient in outpatient clinic in 1 week.

Sharon Weintraub, PharmD

Answers for Jerome's Case

1. a. Information from the chart: history of present illness; full medication history; compliance history; full social history; past medical history relevant to psychiatric illness; results of physical exam; results of psychiatric and mental status admission exams; laboratory results relevant to psychiatric admission and medication use—electrolytes, basic chemistries, renal/hepatic function, thyroid function tests, venereal disease tests.

   b. Information from Jerome: subjective description of chief complaint; subjective response to previous drug therapy; subjective reports of perceived adverse drug reactions; social history especially as it affects medication taking behavior; compliance history; drug samples, nonprescription medications, nutritional supplements and herbal products used; history of substance abuse and readiness to quit if positive history; history of suicide attempts; patient's desired outcome for this admission and for drug therapy and preferred means to achieve those outcomes; information from wife or other caregivers on most of this same information, depending on patient's ability to respond to questions clearly and accurately.

2. a. Inappropriate compliance: either cannot afford or prefers not to take valproate and lithium (actual problem—serum levels are below detectable limits—serious and acute, Priority 1).

b. Inappropriate compliance: either cannot afford or prefers not to take paroxetine (potential problem—no positive evidence that it exists but have high index of suspicion due to poor compliance with other medications—serious and acute, Priority 1).

c. Needs additional drug therapy: untreated condition of tobacco and substance abuse (actual problem; serious, not acute; Priority 3).

3. a. Inappropriate compliance with valproate, lithium and paroxetine: The patient will demonstrate an understanding of the importance of medication compliance in his illness and will take/refill his medication correctly at least 80% of the time. Target serum lithium level 0.8 to 1mEq/L. Target total serum valproate level 60mcg/mL.

b. Needs additional drug therapy: The patient will demonstrate an understanding of the harmful effects of substance abuse on his illness and will enroll in stop-smoking program and discontinue marijuana use after discharge from hospital.

4. a. Inappropriate compliance with valproate, lithium and paroxetine: Provide a medication reminder box to patient; or provide extensive patient counseling to both patient and spouse.

b. Needs additional drug therapy: Enroll patient in smoking and substance abuse programs; or perform complete patient work-up on readiness to change behaviors using Transtheoretical Model for Change.

5. a. Inappropriate compliance with valproate, lithium and paroxetine: Provide extensive patient education to patient and spouse. Discuss pathophysiology of his illness and importance of medication in controlling symptoms. Discuss consequences of poor compliance. Discuss compliance strategies such as pill boxes, dosing calendars, etc. and provide the preferred tool to patient. Discuss adverse effect monitoring and risk/benefit of drug therapy and disease state. Discuss strategies for managing missed doses.

b. Needs additional therapy: Evaluate patient's readiness for change. If not at planning or later state, provide general educational materials and follow up in 1 month to repeat evaluation. If at planning or later state, discuss smoking cessation options with patient (patch, gum, bupropion) and help obtain necessary smoking-cessation aid. Monitor patient weekly for progress. If at planning or later stage for marijuana use, recommend to physician to refer patient to substance abuse clinic. Patient will be followed in clinic.

c. Monitoring
Inappropriate compliance: Contact patient 1 week after discharge and obtain compliance history. Inquire into any problems he has noted with medication including adverse effects, affordability. If cannot afford medication, enroll in patient assistance program. Monitor medication refill dates x 3 months. Monitor serum levels of valproate (target level 60mcg/mL) and lithium (target level 0.8 to 1 mcg/mL) 1 week after discharge.

Needs additional therapy: Contact patient 1 week after discharge. Ensure he has smoking cessation aids, answer questions, inquire into adverse effects (irritability, vivid dreams), assess if using smoking cessation aid appropriately. Inquire if interested in referral to substance abuse program.

d. Rationale

Inappropriate compliance: Include spouse in discussion. Patient seems too agitated to pay close attention. Consequences of poor compliance in this patient are severe, so must use extensive compliance-related education.

Needs additional therapy: patient may not be ready to quit smoking or illicit drug use. Will only be able to intervene with hope of success if patient is at the planning or later stage of readiness for change.

6. Most of these interventions are patient-focused. Need to ensure that Jerome and his spouse understand the importance of medication and the consequences of poor compliance, and that they agree to make sure he takes his medication correctly. If he is willing to quit smoking, unless he wishes to use bupropion, the care plan can be implemented by working with both the patient and his spouse. Need to ensure they understand which product to obtain, which strength to buy, how to use/apply the product, its common side effects, how to taper the dose, and what to do in case Jerome still smokes while trying to quit. If he prefers to use bupropion, the pharmacist will need to discuss getting a prescription from the physician. Similarly, the pharmacist will need to work with the physician to obtain a referral to a substance abuse clinic if Jerome wishes to stop smoking marijuana.

7. Drug therapy problems: inappropriate compliance with valproate, lithium, and paroxetine; needs additional drug therapy for smoking cessation and substance abuse.

S: Performed intake medication history on this 24-year-old male with recent onset of mania. He has a 2-year history of bipolar affective disorder managed with lithium carbonate 300 mg po bid, valproic acid sustained release 500 mg po tid and paroxetine 20 mg po qd. Risperidone 2 mg qhs, repeat x 1 prn added while in hospital. Has positive history for tobacco and cannabis use.

O: Serum lithium and valproate levels on admission were below detectable limits. Na 132 mEq/L. Remaining chemistries non-contributory.

A: Patient demonstrates poor medication compliance with lithium and valproate. Must assume compliance with paroxetine is also poor. Medication noncompliance likely a precipitating factor in this current admission. History is positive for tobacco and cannabis abuse.

P: Will provide extensive medication education to patient and spouse with hope that spouse may be able to assist patient with medication taking. Will provide dosing calendar and/or pill reminder box as per patient preference. Will assess patient's readiness to stop smoking and enter substance abuse program. If ready to change, will assist patient with obtaining appropriate smoking cessation aid and provide smoking cessation education. If wishes referral to substance abuse clinic, will request psychiatric team for referral. Will contact patient 1 week after discharge to re-assess compliance and obtain serum valproate and lithium levels. Will monitor medication refill dates x 3 months. If not already referred to substance abuse program after discharge, will re-assess willingness for referral at that time.

Samir Kahn, PharmD

Chapter 9

Answers for Mrs. Corrigan's Case

1.a. Data from the medical record: vital signs; physical exam; lipid panel; diabetes studies (blood glucose, hemoglobin A1c, and urinary protein); anemia studies (CBC, hemoglobin, and hematocrit); renal and hepatic function; basic serum chemistries; bone density screening.

  b. Data from Mrs. Corrigan: subjective descriptions of medical conditions and general health; subjective descriptions of response to medications including perceived adverse drug reactions; social history including financial barriers to health care and medication use; nonprescription, herbal, and nutritional medications used prior to admission; patient preferences for her care.

2.a. Wrong drug: contraindication present for glyburide. Creatinine clearance calculated as 31mL/min. Glyburide relatively contraindicated with creatinine clearance below 50mL/min. (actual; serious, not acute; Priority 3.)

  b. Needs additional drug therapy: requires renal protection for nephropathy in diabetic patient (actual; serious, not acute; Priority 3).

  c. Needs additional drug therapy: pneumococcal vaccine in institutionalized elderly resident (potential pending further history; serious, not acute; Priority 3).

  d. Dosage too low: ferrous sulfate. Hemoglobin and hematocrit remain below normal. (actual; serious, not acute; Priority 3.)

  e. Unnecessary drug: no medical indication for cyanocobalamin and loratidine (potential pending further history; not serious, not acute; Priority 3).

3.a. Wrong drug for glyburide: Patient will receive drug therapy to maintain blood glucose and hemoglobin A1c within clinically appropriate range without suffering adverse drug effects such as hypoglycemia.

b. Needs additional drug therapy for renal protection: Patient will receive appropriate renally protective medication without suffering adverse drug effects such as hyperkalemia, cough, or hypotension.

c. Needs additional drug therapy with pneumococcal vaccine: Patient will receive all medically indicated vaccines without suffering adverse drug effects.

d. Dosage too low for ferrous sulfate: Patient will receive therapeutic dose of ferrous sulfate. Hemoglobin and hematocrit will increase to normal range and patient will not suffer adverse drug reactions such as gastric upset or constipation.

e. Unnecessary drug therapy for cyanocobalamin and loratidine: Patient will not receive medically non-indicated medication and will not suffer relapse or worsening of any previous illness or disease state.

4. a. Wrong drug for glyburide: switch glyburide to glipizide 5 mg qd; switch glyburide to rosiglitazone 4 mg qd.

b. Needs additional therapy for renal protection: add lisinopril 5 mg qd; add irbesartan 150 mg qd.

c. Needs additional drug therapy with pneumococcal vaccine: administer pneumococcal vaccine x 1; verify vaccination history with patient and/or physician prior to vaccine administration.

d. Dosage too low for ferrous sulfate: increase dose to 325 mg bid; maintain 325 mg qd dose and monitor.

e. Unnecessary drug therapy for loratidine and cyanocobalamin: discontinue medications; verify lack of indication with physician prior to discontinuing medications.

5. a. Wrong drug for glyburide: Discontinue glyburide, start glipizide at 5 mg qd and increase dose as indicated by blood glucose to maximum 20 mg qd. Patient has already responded to sulfonylurea therapy, so prefer that to rosiglitazone. Patient had previous edema from pioglitazone. Monitor blood glucose daily until adequate response achieved, then twice weekly. Monitor hemoglobin A1c q 3 months.

b. Needs additional therapy for renal protection: Start irbesartan 150 mg qd and increase to maximum of 300 mg qd as tolerated. Patient had previous hyperkalemia on fosinopril, so prefer different class of medication. Monitor blood pressure daily x 1 week then monthly. Monitor electrolytes in 1 week, then monthly x 3 months. Monitor cough.

c. Needs additional drug therapy with pneumococcal vaccine: Contact primary care provider and request vaccination history. If vaccine not given, administer x 1. Monitor for adverse effects.

d. Dosage too low for ferrous sulfate: Increase ferrous sulfate to bid. Patient is still anemic and no complaints of intolerance to iron to date. Monitor hemoglobin and hematocrit in 2 weeks, then q 3 months. Monitor for constipation, gastric intolerance.

e. Unnecessary drug therapy for loratidine and cyanocobalamin: Contact physician and verify indication. If none, recommend discontinue both medications. Will not discontinue at this time in case lack of indication is only a documentation problem. Monitor allergy signs and symptoms x 1 week. Obtain CBC with iron studies. If MCV increased, re-evaluate if cyanocobalamin may be indicated and restart at that time.

6. Implementation of care plan primarily requires cooperation of physician. Pharmacist must request that glyburide be discontinued, new orders for glipizide and irbesartan be written, and dosage of ferrous sulfate be increased. Pharmacist must request additional information from primary care physician concerning indications for pneumococcal vaccine, loratidine, and cyanocobalamin. Depending on results, new orders to administer or discontinue those medications must be written. Nursing staff should be apprised of new medications and changes in existing ones. Mrs. Corrigan should receive patient counseling on her medication changes and be informed of the reason for the medication changes, the monitoring plan, and any adverse effects for which she can self-monitor.

7. Drug Therapy Problems: wrong drug (glyburide); needs additional therapy (renal protection); needs additional drug therapy (pneumococcal vaccine); dosage too low (ferrous sulfate); unnecessary drug therapy (loratidine and cyanocobalamin).

S: Admission Drug Regimen Review performed today for new resident, Mrs. Roberta Corrigan. Resident is 70-year-old woman with a history of Type 2 diabetes mellitus, diabetic nephropathy, hypertension, peripheral vascular disease, iron deficiency anemia, hyperlipidemia, and osteoporosis. Current medication list consists of simvastatin 40 mg qd, hydrochlorothiazide 25 mg qd, glyburide 10 mg bid, oyster calcium 500 mg bid, alendronate 70 mg q Monday, amlodipine 10 mg qd, nabumetone 500 mg bid, cyanocobalamin 1000 mcg IM qmonthly, ferrous sulfate 325 mg qd, loratidine 10 mg qd, influenza vaccine on admission. Patient voices no complaints concerning her medications and states she generally feels well. Previous medication sensitivities/adverse effect include metformin (diarrhea), pioglitazone (edema), and fosinopril (hyperkalemia).

O: All results from admission exam by Dr. Connors.
Vital Signs: BP 138/80; HR 100, RR 12, T 98.8.
Lipids: Within normal limits.
Chemistries: Within normal limits except BUN 21 mg/dL, Cr 1.4 mg/dL, Creatinine Clearance calculated as 31mL/min, Random glucose 138 mg/dL, Hemoglobin A1c 7.3%, Urinary protein 16mg/dL.
Hematology: Within normal limits except Hemoglobin 10.2g/L, Hematocrit 30.8%, Serum Iron 48 mcg/dL, Total Iron Binding Capacity 460 mcg/dL.

A: Glyburide is relatively contraindicated with a creatinine clearance of < 50mL/min. Patient has modest proteinuria and requires renally protective medication to prevent worsening. Dosage of ferrous sulfate too low (patient still anemic). Vaccination status not complete (patient may require pneumococcal vaccine). Indications for loratidine and cyanocobalamin unclear and must be verified.

P: Suggest the following: d/c glyburide and start glipizide 5 mg qd and taper up according to blood glucose. Monitor blood glucose daily until adequate response achieved, then twice weekly. Monitor hemoglobin A1c q 3 months.

Start irbesartan 150 mg qd and taper up to 300 mg qd as tolerated. Monitor blood pressure daily x 1 week then monthly. Monitor electrolytes in 1 week, then monthly x 3 months. Monitor cough.

Increase ferrous sulfate to 325 mg bid. Monitor hemoglobin and hematocrit in 2 weeks, then q 3 months. Monitor for constipation, gastric intolerance.

Confirm vaccination history with Dr. Connor and administer pneumococcal vaccine if not previously administered. Verify indications for loratidine and cyanocobalamin with Dr. Connor. D/C if no longer indicated. Monitor for relapse of any previous signs/symptoms of allergy or macrocytic anemia.

Ken Schwartz, RPh, CGP

Answers for Mr. Hensler's Case

1. a. Data from the medical record: any new/recent objective data that demonstrates therapeutic or adverse drug effects including thyroid function tests, blood glucose, Hemoglobin A1c, electroylytes, complete blood count, liver function tests, renal function tests. Physician's history and physical that demonstrates therapeutic or adverse drug effects, dermatological exam, musculoskeletal exam, neurological exam. Vital signs.

   b. Data from Mr. Hensler: subjective descriptions of medical conditions and general health; subjective descriptions of response to medications including perceived adverse drug reactions.

2. Adverse drug reaction: undesirable effect of hepatotoxicity caused by atorvastatin.

3. The patient's blood lipids will be maintained at the recommended levels without resulting in adverse effects of drug therapy.

4. Start ezetimibe 10 mg qd; start colesevelam 3 tablets bid.

5. Start ezetimibe 10 mg qd. Only needs to be taken once daily and has modestly beneficial effects on HDL levels in addition to lowering total cholesterol, LDL, and triglycerides. Monitor serum lipid profile in 1 month. Monitor for adverse effects including headache, myalgias, rash, pancreatitis.

6. Care plan will be implemented by contacting physician and recommending addition of ezetimibe. Mr. Hensler needs to be counseled on the medication change, the reason it happened, the monitoring tests he can expect, and adverse effects for which he can self-monitor.

7. Drug therapy problem: adverse drug reaction.

S: Atorvastatin therapy discontinued in this 85-year-old resident due to significant increase in liver function tests. Has long-standing history of hyperlipidemia previously well controlled on atorvastatin 20 mg qd. Resident voices no complaints with drug therapy and did not notice any changes in skin color, urine, or stools. Remainder of drug therapy and medical problem list is unchanged and stable.

O: Lipid profile from 6/20/this year: Total cholesterol 188mg/dL, HDL 44mg/dL, LDL 88mg/dL, Triglycerides 133mg/dL.
Liver function tests from 9/21/this year: ALT 288U/L, AST 302U/L, Alkaline. Phosphatase 249U/L, Total bilirubin 0.7 mg/dL, Prothrombin time 12 seconds.

A: Adverse drug reaction to atorvastatin resulting in hepatotoxicity. Resident requires new therapy for existing hyperlipidemia.

P: Suggest start ezetimibe 10 mg qd. Repeat lipid profile in 1 month. Will re-evaluate during next month's drug regimen review.

Kathy Kloster, PharmD

Chapter 10
Answers for Fred's Case
1.a. Information from the chart: patient demographics; history of present illness, how long he has had diabetes, what degree of control was present, what education has been given and when, treatment goals established, plan for further evaluation, care and education from the last visit, full medication history; previous vital signs and results of physician's physical examination; laboratory parameters for diabetes control and for target organ damage; past medical history; social, family, and other information that might affect ability to achieve outcomes.

b. Information from Fred: patient's assessment of chief complaint (given above); expanded information on what he is doing for altering food intake; detailed history of how actually taking medications, confirming all prescription, nonprescription, and alternative medication; home blood glucose monitoring results; perceived difficulties in adhering to treatment plan.

2. a. Inappropriate compliance: patient unable to take metformin as written (actual, Priority 1).

b. Inappropriate compliance: patient unable to make dietary modifications (actual, Priority 2).

c. Needs additional drug therapy: low HDL and elevated triglycerides may need to be treated (potential, Priority 3).

3. a. Slow progression of diabetes complication by keeping FBG 90-130 mg/dL Post Prandial BG < 180 mg/dL and HgA1c < 7.0%.

b. Slow the progress of dyslipidemia complications by keeping HDL > 40 mg/dL and triglycerides < 150 mg/dL.

c. Slow the progress of hypertension complications by keeping BP < 130/80 mmHg.

d. Slow the progress of cardiovascular complications by maintaining healthy body weight with Body Mass Index (BMI) < 25.

4. a. Diabetes: Metformin, work with patient to find triggers in daily activities to take medication BID, switch patient to QD dosage form 1000 mg/day (Glucophage XR).

b. Dietary Intervention: Discuss with dietitian, track in small interventions with diet more specific to what actually eating, have patient keep food diary of all foods eaten, perform diet diagnosis to help patient make smart food choices, educate on increasing vegetables, free foods and portion control.

c. Dyslipidemia: Dietary recommendation above, recheck lipids in 6 months, recheck lipids once blood glucose under control, do nothing. Lipids are likely to be uncontrolled in an uncontrolled diabetic, recommend starting triglyceride lowering agent such as gemfibrozil 600 mg BID.

5. Therapeutic plan:
   a. Change prescription to Glucophage XR 1000 mg with evening meal. Follow up with patient in 2 weeks to check blood glucose and assess compliance with new dosage form. Recheck HgA1c in 3 months.

   b. Have patient keep food diary for 1 month. Follow up with diabetes educator or pharmacist regarding diet changes in 1 month.

c. Dietary recommendations from dietician and pharmacist. Recheck lipids in 6 months to determine need for drug therapy.

6. Implementation Plan:
   a. Have staff physician (Dr. Jones) write Rx for Glucophage XR 500 mg, 2 tablets at evening meal, # 60, 2 refills.

   b. Give patient basic food diary sheets and instruct him to keep record of all food and beverages consumed for next month. Have patient make appointment for follow up with me in 28 days.

   c. Reinforce initial dietary recommendations, counsel patient on completing food diary so can give specific recommendations in 1 month

7. Fred Willert 10/23/06.
   Inappropriate compliance: patient unable to take metformin as written.
   Inappropriate compliance: patient unable to make dietary modifications.

S: Fred presents today for first follow-up visit after diagnosis on 9/12 and initial visit 9/22. He was started on metformin 500 mg BID. Fred states that he gets up late and frequently doesn't eat breakfast and so doesn't take his metformin in the morning. He doesn't take it when he is at work for lunch and often gets home late for the evening meal and doesn't take it then either. Best estimate is 6 doses taken in last month. Dietary changes are also an issue, especially scheduling and portion sizes. He is adjusting to the diagnosis and is committed to continue trying, but realizes he has work to do. He cannot afford another session with dietitians.

O: BP 132/80 mm Hg, Wt. 236 lbs, Ht. 5'7", BMI 36.9, Fasting BG 138 mg/dL.

A: Fred is not yet able to adjust to adding new medication and dietary changes to his life over the last month. Minimal compliance is limiting therapy results.

P: Recommended to Dr. Jones switching to Glucophage XR 2 x 500 mg tablets with evening meal. Rx written for #60 with 2 refills. Counseled patient to discontinue current metformin and begin once daily medication. Fred agreed to work on routinely eating an evening meal and taking his medication. Fred agreed to work with me on simple dietary changes and will complete a food diary for the next month.

F/U: I will call patient at home in 2 weeks to assess compliance and blood glucose progress to FBG < 130mg/dL and PPBG < 180 mg/dL. Pt. will return to clinic in 1 month, assess food diary, med compliance, and blood glucose values. Recheck HbA1c in 3 months.

Sue Mason, PharmD

10/23/06 Needs additional drug therapy, low HDL and elevated Triglycerides may need to be treated

S: Fred returned to the clinic today where diabetes and previous laboratory results were reviewed. Recently diagnosed with Type 2 diabetes and hypertension. Has been on treatment approx 1 month. No previous knowledge of lipid disorder. He smokes > 20 cigarettes per day and has about 10 alcoholic drinks per week. Mother with diabetes at 55 y.o., Father with MI at 62 y.o.

O: 10/23/06   BP 132/80 mm Hg, Wt. 236 lbs, Ht. 5'7", BMI 36.9, BG-138 mg/dL.
   09/09/06 Total Cholesterol 176, HDL Chol 34, LDL Chol 93, Triglycerides 245.

A: Patient's low HDL and elevated Triglycerides may require treatment if unresponsive to dietary manipulation in this high-risk man.

P: Encouraged Fred to make slow and steady progress on dietary changes. He is completing food diary for DM diet. Will address tobacco and ethanol in future visits.

F/U: Pt. to return to clinic in one month. Assess food diary, HBGM values identify dietary challenges, assess willingness to consider smoking cessation. Repeat fasting lipid panel in 6 months.

Sue Mason, PharmD

Answers for Allison's Case

1.a. Because this is a patient you see frequently, you already have a complete medical and medication history for this patient. At this visit, you want to assess patient compliance with taking warfarin and other medications. It is important to document any changes in medications, including nonprescription and herbal medications. For this case, diet is important because warfarin interacts with several foods. In addition to the information you collect from the patient, you would refer to the patient record for information documented up to and including the last visit.

2.a. Dose too low: drug interaction with diet high in leafy green vegetables. Warfarin INR 1.7 outside recommended range of 2.0-3.0 (actual, Priority 1.)

   b. Drug use without indication: "unknown" diet medication (potential, Priority 2).

3.a. atrial fibrillation: Prevent clot formation by maintaining INR of 2.5 (goal 2.0-3.0) for anticoagulation therapy.

   b. hypertension: Slow the progress of hypertension complications by keeping BP < 140/90 mmHg.

c. overweight status: Slow the progress of cardiovascular complications by maintaining healthy body weight with Body Mass Index (BMI) < 25.

4. a. Increase warfarin dose and recheck INR in one week, remain on same dose. Counsel patient on the importance of eating consistent diet. Counsel patient on foods that interact with warfarin (foods high in Vitamin K).

   b. Discontinue herbal diet medication. Bring in bottle of medication to clinic to determine efficacy and safety. Encourage therapeutic lifestyle changes (increased exercise and decreased calories) to lose weight.

5. Therapeutic plan:
   a. Since Allison wants to continue with her dietary changes, increase warfarin dose by approximately 10% to increase INR from 1.7 to 2.0 (current dose 35 mg/wk, new dose 37.5 mg/wk) by giving 1 ½ tablets (7.5 mg) on Mondays. Counsel patient on importance of eating consistent diet and let her know if she discontinues diet high in Vitamin K her INR will increase. Recheck INR in one week.

   b. Call clinic with name and ingredients in herbal product. Discontinue herbal diet medication if any ingredients interact with warfarin or efficacy for product has not been established through randomized controlled trials. Continue therapeutic lifestyle changes to decrease weight 1-2 pounds per week. Patient will document weight at next clinic visit in 1 week.

6. Implementation plan:
   a. Allison already has the warfarin 5 mg tablets, and since not adding any new strengths will instruct her on the change in dosage on Mondays both verbally and in writing. Will counsel her on maintaining a consistent intake of leafy green vegetables and give her a handout on vegetables with significant Vitamin K.

   b. Counsel her to discontinue the herbal diet medication and not add any medications (nonprescription, vitamins, herbals) without first contacting the clinic. Encourage her to continue caloric restriction and moderate exercise with goal to lose 1-2 pounds per week.

7. Allison Chance 10/23/06
   Dose too low: drug interaction with diet high in leafy green vegetables and warfarin. Drug use without indication: "unknown" diet medication.

S: Allison presents today for routine monthly warfarin management appt. She is currently taking warfarin 5 mg/day (35 mg/week) as directed, no other Rx or nonprescription medication changes. She states she started a diet 2 weeks ago and has increased her intake of leafy green vegetables. She wants to continue with dietary changes. She also added an herbal diet preparation, but is unsure of its name or its ingredients. No other complaints.

O: BP 120/78 mm Hg, Pulse 66 bpm irregular, Wt. 178 lbs, Ht. 5'8", INR-1.7.

A: Increase in leafy green vegetable intake (vit K) likely cause for drop in INR. Unknown herbal product may also affect INR and unlikely to be effective in assisting in weight loss.

P: Increase warfarin dose by approx. 10%. Instructed Allison to increase from 35 mg/week to 37.5 mg/week by adding ½ tablet (total of 7.5 mg) on Monday. Changes made to patient's dosage calendar. Counseled Allison on the importance of maintaining consistent vitamin K intake in diet to allow for accurate dosing of warfarin, and to not add make changes in meds, diet, or supplements without telling us. Gave her the vegetable/vitamin K handout. Instructed Allison to contact the clinic with the name and ingredients of supplement and will recommend it be discontinued if any ingredients interact with warfarin or efficacy for product has not been established through randomized controlled trials. Reinforced decreased caloric intake and increased exercise. She agreed to contact us if her diet changed.

F/U: Return to clinic in one week for recheck of INR to assure adequate prevention with INR ≥ 2.0, assess for bleeding, weight, and dietary changes. Allison to contact us with changes before then.

Elliott Regan, PharmD

Index

F

F/U (follow-up) section, of SOAP note plan, 157–158
Faxes. *See* Letters
Flow sheets, 147–148
    sample, 149f
Follow-up monitoring, 25f, 26. *See also* Monitoring
    documentation of, 140, 150t
    in DRR *vs.* pharmaceutical care, 180
    of patient care plans, 128–133
        patient-focused, 122, 123–124
    in SOAP note plan (F/U section), 157–158,
        159–160

G

Geriatric Pharmacotherapy Monitoring Form, 60,
    69f–70f
Goals, therapeutic. *See* Therapeutic goals

H

Hagel, H., 29
Health care system, drug therapy problems in, 9–10,
    121
Health Insurance Portability and Accountability Act
    (HIPAA), 51, 74
Health status data, 76
Health system pharmacy. *See* Hospital pharmacy
Hepler, Charles, 5, 6t, 7
Herbal supplements, 10
History taking. *See* Patient data collection; Patient
    interview
Hospital pharmacy, 169–172
    adverse drug reaction monitoring in, 13, 170
    case studies, 172–176
    common clinical services in, 169–170
    medication reconciliation in, 40, 170
    and nursing facility practice, 178
Hospitalizations, 9, 10
Hospitalized patients
    discharged, 10, 40, 94
    monitoring form for, 60, 67f–68f
Hospitals, requesting patient data from, 75

I

Inappropriate compliance. *See* Noncompliance
Indications. *See also* "Appropriate indication";
    "Untreated indications"
    unapproved, 101
"Ineffective drug." *See* "Wrong drug"
Inpatient pharmacy. *See* Hospital pharmacy

Institute of Medicine (IOM)
    on medication errors, 9, 13–14
    on patient safety, 9, 13
Interventions
    'do nothing,' 119
    drug-focused, 118–119
    patient-focused, 117–118
    by pharmacist, documentation of, 139, 140

J

Johnson, J. A., 11
Joint Commission of Pharmacy Practitioners, 15
Joint Commission on Accreditation of Healthcare
    Organizations (JCAHO), 40

K

*Knowledge Coupling: New Premises and New Tools for
Medical Care and Education* (Weed), 157–158

L

Laboratory data, 49, 50
    in clinics and ambulatory settings, 189
    in long-term-care settings, 178
    requesting, 75
LDL cholesterol levels, 12
Leading questions, 55
Letters
    in patient chart, 151
    to physician, on drug-focused care plan, 125–126,
        127–128
        example, 228–229
Lifestyle-related care plans, 122
Listening, 57
Long-term-care pharmacy, 177–181
    case studies, 182–184
    Drug Regimen Review (DRR) in, 178–181
    patient monitoring form for, 60, 69f–70f

M

Mail-order pharmacy, 15
Medical diagnosis, 41
Medical history, 77–78
Medical problems
    and drug therapy problems, 26–27
    list in patient chart, 146f, 147
Medicare Part D, 14–15, 180. *See also* Medication
    Therapy Management Services (MTMS)
Medication education, in hospital pharmacy, 170